DENTAL PRACTICE HERO

FROM ORDINARY PRACTICE TO EXTRAORDINARY EXPERIENCE

Dental Practice Hero

From Ordinary Practice to Extraordinary Experience

ACKNOWLEDGMENTS

I'd like to thank all the greats in dentistry and business that have helped me on my journey of developing the ideas in this book. I have read so many books and been to so many seminars, that it is often difficult to remember where the information came from. I started my dental career with a strong conviction that "success leaves clues." That alone has allowed me to take so many pearls from many educators and blend them into my own.

In no particular order, Scott Leune who gave me the confidence to take a risk and scratch start a practice. Bruce Baird, Vicky Mcmanus, Steve Rasner, David Hornbrook, and Paul Homoly who helped me with verbiage and treatment presentation and taught me that the only thing holding my practice back was myself. The clinical gurus: Bill Strupp, Frank Spears, Peter Dawson, Carl Misch, Cliff Ruddle, Tommy Murph, Gayle Fletcher, Arun Garg, and Brock Rondeau. All the doctors and consultants on the podcast circuits, especially Mark Costes, Gary Takacs, David Maloley, Howard Farran, and Alan Mead.

All the other people who have contributed to the profession and allowed dentists to take dentistry to new heights.

My early mentors Stephen Zeck and Rene Tanquilit.

My parents, who raised me to be who I am today. The values and beliefs I hold are a direct result of your love.

All the people at Nelson Ridge Family Dental: Justine, Lauren, Joanna, Amy, Jaclyn, Pam, Amanda, Kristie, Andrea, Kathy,

Calla, Ashley, Vicky, Krista, and Corrie. You girls took the vision and made it a reality.

Most of all, my amazing wife, Joanna, who has stood by me since we started dating in high school. I could never have reached the heights I did without your support and love.

Last, I dedicate this book to my daughters, Briella and Alyssa, in hopes that one day when you are older I can teach you firsthand what a great profession dentistry is.

TABLE OF CONTENTS

INTRODUCTION
AN ADVENTURE WAITING TO HAPPEN

People are made to make stories. We all tell ourselves stories about our lives and the lives of the people around us. Sometimes, our story is the stereotypical success story. "I started out with nothing, worked hard, and now I'm at the top of my field." Most of the time, our story is less satisfying. "I had dreams, but they're dead now, and I just slog through my days." "It's never getting better. I just have to keep on going until I'm dead or retire."

I'm here to tell you that a different story is possible for you and your practice. Your dental practice is an adventure in the making, and you are a heroic dentist about to begin a quest to create an epic practice that your patients, employees, and most importantly, you and your family, will love. It starts with a quick trip back to the beginning, when you were not yet the dentist you've become.

An Apprentice Looks at His Life

When did you decide that you wanted to be a dentist? I'm sure you wrote the answer as part of your entrance essay to get into dental school, but was it the truth? Let's be honest. For most of us, dentistry wasn't always our dream. And later down the line, once we became dentists, it wasn't our "dream come true" either.

What were your expectations about the life you would lead once you were a dentist? Are you meeting them? Were angry patients, staff issues, failed restorations, and negative Google reviews part of your dream? Were PPO write offs and the growing corporate penetration part of it too? These are the realities we live with in our current dental landscape, and they aren't changing. Dentistry is stressful. I want to repeat that: dentistry is STRESSFUL! I know because I am a dentist and I talk to other dentists all of the time. I have yet to meet one that says, "Ain't it great? I drill a little hole in a tooth and shove some goop in there with my thumb and they pay me an insane amount of money to do it!"

The reality is that what we do day in, day out is difficult work. It's hard on our bodies and even harder on our mental state. It takes immense amounts of concentration and often frustration. We work in a difficult environment. Pile that up with running a business, staff issues, paying the bills, and trying to maintain a good work-life balance, and you can see why many of our colleagues are disappointed with their choice of a profession.

I want you to go back to when you were young and you could dream, but this time, I want you to dream forward from where you are now in the present. I want you to think about what your epic practice would be like. How you would feel if you had it? What it would do for your life and your family?

Next, I want to tell you that you can have it. This is not pie-in-the-sky thinking; I really mean it. You already have all the skills, you have the resources, and hopefully since you are reading this book, you have the motivation.

And contrary to what you might think, I am going to tell you it's easy.

When I really think about it, it's incredibly easy. It just takes a new way of thinking about the way you run your business, and a bit of applying the skills you have to a new area of your life. I want you to be the hero of your practice, leaping over obstacles at your practice and slaying the monsters that try to defeat you. I want you to work the days and hours you want to, be highly compensated for it, and most of all, love every minute of it.

I want your life to be fun again, and for you to enter each day not as a poor schlub slogging through the demands of his practice, but as a hero, using your unique powers to improve patient lives and experiences while reaping great rewards. Together, we can rewrite the story of your life and your career so that it's fun again. You can be a hero to your patients and your staff while loving what you do.

Your Heroic Journey

Have you ever noticed that most books and movies have essentially the same plot? Anthropologists tell us that's because there are only seven basic stories in the world. These story-forms are universal and cross-cultural. They're part of being human and they're how people make sense of the world.

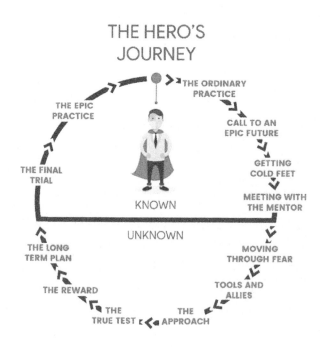

THE HERO'S JOURNEY

One of the most basic human stories—one that occurs in every culture, time, and place—is the story of the Hero's Journey. It's the tale of someone who takes a journey from their everyday world to an unknown land, in search of a great treasure. The hero returns home, but is forever changed by the journey, and home is no longer the boring place he left behind. His adventures have transformed him from everyman into an epic hero, and he, in turn, changes the world around him.

I'm going to tell you a new story that takes the form of a hero's journey. It is the story of a hero, chosen from an ordinary life and sent on a fantastic quest. He puts together a team of sidekicks, chooses his magical weapons, defeats all obstacles, and wins the greatest prize of all.

But this hero is unusual. His sidekicks answer phones and clean teeth. His magical weapons include loupes, handpieces, and burrs. And he doesn't wear armor, he wears a shirt and tie. This hero is a dentist, and the prize for his labors is a thriving, fulfilling independent practice where he can change lives while loving his work. Welcome to the world of heroic dentistry. You're about to embark on the journey of a lifetime.

Note: Get a pen and notebook ready, because throughout this book we're going to be setting goals, making plans, and coming up with the next actionable steps. It's not enough to do this in your head. It's not enough to type yourself a note on your phone. You have to write it down. Studies have shown that written goals solidify commitment, enhance problem solving, and increase follow-through. It's not pop psychology, it's human nature. *You have to write it down.*

CHAPTER 1
THE ORDINARY PRACTICE

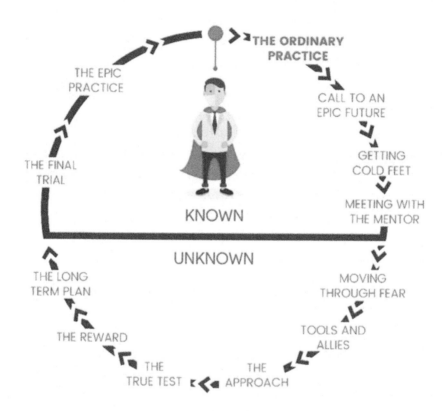

Every hero has to start somewhere. Before King Arthur could pull the sword from the stone and build up Camelot, he had to serve as a squire in the house of Sir Ector. Before Mario was leaping over mushrooms and searching for princesses, he was a plumber. Batman began as little Bruce, walking home from the theater safe between his parents. Until you have a clear sense of where you are right now, you can't really envision the goal of your journey.

It's time to take a good, hard look at your life and your career. Once you understand what your ordinary is like, you can prepare to leave it behind and start training to be a hero.

An Unexpected Practice

When you started dental school, you probably imagined a relaxing future in an independent practice. You'd have a real connection to your town or neighborhood. You'd see patients, help improve their lives, and have plenty of time for your hobbies and your family. You'd never have to worry about money, and you'd spend most of your time and mental effort 'doing dentistry.'

And then, reality hit.

You're suddenly at the helm of a hectic small business. There are taxes and regulations. People expect you to make decisions about HR and marketing. Even 'doing dentistry' isn't as simple as you imagined. Patients don't always want to pay for treatments, you're constantly balancing their needs against the demands of their insurance, and that corporate practice across town has recalibrated everyone's idea of what dentistry should cost them.

Everything is constantly in flux, and you're not really sure what the future holds. You just know that it's going to be a battle to get from here to there.

Looming Challenges

Corporate dentistry and increased insurance penetration are changing the very nature of our world. A 2012 study found that 69% of patients cite being in-network for dental insurance as important or very important[1]. As certain insurers gain larger shares in the market, they're using their position to force down prices and dramatically decrease our earnings. When over half of your patient base has a single insurance provider, you can't just drop the provider and go out of network without affecting your patients and their health, and insurers know that.

In response, dentistry has become a volume game. We are forced to work harder and see more and more patients per day, only to take home the same or even less than we did a decade ago. I hear from older dentists all the time about the golden age of dentistry in the 70's and 80's, when all you had to do to be successful was just "open your doors and hang your shingle."

Shakespeare said, "When the sea was calm; all boats alike showed mastership in floating." I hate to break it to you, but the seas are not calm anymore. If we keep hoping for the golden age to come back, we will drown. We must learn to ride the new and tumultuous tide.

Many dentists fear that corporate dentistry will forever change the way they practice. If anything, I feel that corporate has shown us an example of how to be better at taking care of people. We have to accommodate our patients, give them excellent experiences, and realize that they're consumers who can make choices about where they receive dental care. Corporate practices are there to make a profit, and they know how to do it. They will always have lower supply and lab costs due to their negotiating strengths. They will also have better in-network fee schedules, due to their size. They will have late hours, Saturday hours, convenient payment plans, and the latest technology, because that's where they put their focus.

So how is a single-owner, private practice to compete? I'll tell you exactly how—by creating such a great patient experience, that people will be willing to accept the lack of convenience as a tradeoff for the outstanding care that they receive. Patient experience (PX) is how you can beat corporate dentistry and thrive in the new economy. The other option is to work until 8 or 9 PM each night and be open on Saturdays, all the while taking every PPO known to man. Essentially, you have to become corporate. That is not my idea of an epic practice.

One great advantage that private practice dentists have is our ability to build long-standing relationships between the patient, the dentist, and a stable staff. People would rather see the same dentist and staff every six months than get lost in the revolving door of associates and employees that is a plague for corporations.

Ultimately, corporate is a blessing for the industry. Not only does it help to get more people the care they need, but it also helps us see what an epic practice is not. There is a paradigm shift happening right now. Dental practices need heroic leadership. Those that try to remain ordinary will die.

My goal is for your practice to be different. I want your practice to thrive in any economy, just like mine does. As Spencer Johnson explains in his book *Who Moved My Cheese*, "The quicker you let go of old cheese, the sooner you find new cheese." The dental world has changed. There's no sense clinging to the past. It's time to let go and find a new reality. And that's going to take a hero, a journey, and an epic battle.

My Adventure in Dentistry

The journey starts with a basic premise: that dentistry is a great profession. Do you believe that? You should. Let's think about it a little. A lot of dentists I have talked to have said that they were either going to go into medical or dental; I had that dilemma as well.

I started out in undergrad majoring in economics. I really didn't know what I wanted to do. None of my friends were thinking about dentistry and I didn't have a family member that was already a dentist. I really wanted to be an advertising executive, doing creative marketing campaigns, pitching them in a fancy room with a long conference table, and then calling my wife to tell her how I landed some huge account while talking on my cell phone in my luxury car. I would be wearing a suit. I would be powerful and well respected.

That was my plan.

My junior year I switched majors from economics to advertising. At the University of Illinois Urbana-Champaign, the advertising program was very difficult to get into. I had the grades, and thankfully, I got accepted. I had a family friend who was friends with someone higher up at Leo Burnette Advertising Agency in Chicago. He was going to pull some strings and get me a summer internship.

"Perfect!" I thought. Everything was falling into line.

Unfortunately, the person at the ad agency had a stroke. He left work and went on disability. He no longer could get me the internship I was counting on. The change of plans really took the wind out of my sails. I felt lost. When I looked for different internships online, everyone wanted essays, volunteer experiences, etc. Other than my grades and my personality, I had nothing that made me stand out from the crowd. I could not write an essay for the life of me and I had no experiences that would help me win an internship.

I started thinking about what I'd do if I didn't end up doing the creative side of advertising, which is essentially coming up with the ideas for the campaigns. What if I was stuck writing copy for the rest of my life? What if I was only making $40, 50, or 60k a year? I could never afford that luxury car.

I was the humble son of a carpenter, but I wanted to move up the economic ladder. I wanted prestige. I wanted respect. I had good grades. I knew it was possible to be a physician, but I was slightly turned off by the amount of school. I thought about working in an ER. The idea of someone dying on me because of something I goofed up really scared me. It was at that moment I started thinking about being a dentist.

Truth be told, I hated my dentist.

I hated going to the dentist. I hated the smells, the tastes, everything about it. Yet, I thought, dentists usually only work four days a week, and they make good money. If I really screwed something up, it's only a tooth. I mean, you have so many, how upset could someone be?

I called my Mom one night and told her that I was thinking about dentistry. She was really happy and encouraged me the whole way through. I was already at the end of my junior year at UIUC, so I couldn't switch majors. I had a really rough next two years taking almost 22 credit hours each semester to get in the prerequisites while still majoring in advertising. I graduated, was accepted to the University of Illinois Chicago School of Dentistry, and the rest was history.

I share this story for a reason. Mainly, because I conquered dental school. I never thought I could work so hard. We all did it. We all busted our butts and got the grades so that we could go through four more years of post-graduate training and have this amazing profession. I once heard someone talking about how dental school is a little like the Marines. They beat you down to nothing, get you to rock bottom, then teach you how to work really hard, all to make you a better person.

The big difference is that, unlike the marines, when you get out of dental school, they make it very apparent that you still suck. Dental school breaks us. It makes us feel that if we do everything right in a procedure, the outcome will always be great. If the outcome isn't perfect, it must be our fault. Anyone who knows anything about dentistry will tell you that the teeth are pretty unpredictable animals. Dental school teaches us that when things don't break our way, it's because we broke them.

The Life of a Dentist

So was it all worth it? Let's see. According to the Bureau of Labor Statistics, in 2016, the median dentist earned $159,770 per year[2]. That's a pretty nice salary. Even more so when you think that the people bringing those numbers home are average. That's right, those are average dentists doing dentistry. The BLS says that the best paid earners take home more than $208,000. Even better, I know tons of recent dental school grads working at corporate places taking more than that amount. I understand that the amount of debt dentists are graduating with is rising each year, but still, dentistry pays pretty well.

Let's diverge from average though. I don't want to be an average dentist and I hope you don't either. I want you to crack the top 10%. I believe that if you follow my formula for your practice, you could eventually crack the top 1%, but you will have to put the work in. The top one percent of dentists either make or come pretty close to netting seven figures. How can you argue with that?

I tell you that in every way dentistry is an awesome industry to be in. Let's think about another industry, like golf club sales. How large is their target market? It's mostly men that enjoy golf, but also women. What about the cosmetics industry? Their market consists of women. Practically all of them, about half of the population.

Even better, what about dentistry? Do you know anyone with teeth? Sure you do! Our market is everyone! And even the people without teeth STILL NEED DENTISTRY!!! And when I say "need", I mean they NEED it. People cannot go through life without a dentist. I think, based on this alone, some of the worst dentists in the world can still make a median of $159,770 per year. You can't ask for a better market; it's everybody!

Let's talk about profit margins. We all know that dentistry has one of the highest profit margins across the board. If you don't believe that, look at some other industries. Walmart, for instance, has a 3.1% profit margin[3]. Could you imagine collecting one million dollars one year and only seeing a profit of $31,000 after expenses and payroll? I think we would all hang it up at that point. We enjoy an average around 27%[4]. You can't beat that. And that's average.

It gets even better. In the States, we are protected by the government—through our degrees—from anyone trying to do what we do. Some people down by the border have to deal with dental tourists going down to Mexico, but for most of us, it's a non-issue.

We have very little litigation. I have a friend that is an ER doctor and he couldn't believe I was paying less than five thousand a year for malpractice coverage. Think of what our friends in the medical field are paying. It's nuts!

How about this: I was talking to my wife's OB/GYN before we had our second daughter. He told me there is nothing worse than pulling yourself out of bed at 4AM to deliver a baby. I was telling him about my after hours emergencies: I call in pain meds and an antibiotic and see them on the next day or on Monday if it's a weekend. Who has the harder job?

How about how many hours a week we work? Let's get real here; we've got a good thing going. We make good money and work less than almost everyone else in the nation. We can set our own hours and take as much vacation as we want. Try finding that in other industries.

How great is it that we are licensed to any kind of dentistry we want? You won't find your family doctor taking a weekend course on colonoscopies and then performing them in the office to boost production. Can your OB/GYN go and learn how to do breast augmentation? It would make a lot of sense, since they see a lot of women, but in reality, it just doesn't happen. As a dentist, you can legally do any specialty procedure you want!

If you can't tell, I love this profession. I love what I do. I am a total Continuing Education junky. It drives my wife crazy! I, on average, spend around $20-30k a year on CE. I absolutely love sitting in seminars and learning new things! I love doing all aspects of dentistry! One of the coolest things in the world is taking a tooth from extraction to implant. Or even cooler, taking a broken-down tooth that looks like it can't be saved, doing the endo, bonding a core, and placing a beautiful E-Max crown on it. We get to build things with our hands every day. Dentistry is awesome!

Dentistry Needs Heroes

Finally, the best part about dentistry is that people hate going to the dentist. You read that right. The best part is that people hate us. How many times a day do you hear, "Doc, I just want to you to know I hate the dentist." I hear it at least twice a day, if not more often. According to the American Association of Endodontists, 80% of Americans fear the dentist[5]. Between nine percent and twenty percent of Americans say they avoid going to the dentist because of anxiety or fear, according to dental researcher Peter Milgram, DDS[6]. So why is that so great for us? Why is it a good thing that people hate the dentist? If we get intentional about creating a patient experience that makes them hate going a lot less, they will rave about us. If we make it exceptional, they will be ecstatic. We will be their heroes, because we defeated their fear and pain and created an incredible dental experience.

Every day, my patients tell my staff that we've provided the best dental experience they have ever had. And like I said before, it's easy. Guess who makes it easy? Our colleagues who haven't got a clue how to do it. There are so many bad dental practices in the US that, to stand out, you only have to be slightly nice.

What about corporate practices? I believe they will never be able to replicate what the private dentist can do. They can have great hours and take every insurance, but they can never put the human touch on in the same way we can, as private practice owners. Patients want great care and will pay for it. Consistency is key. Patients want to see the dentist that they trust. The revolving door of corporate associates can never provide that. If you want to compete with corporate, be a dentist that patients love and trust.

This book is about creating a practice that will grow explosively from word of mouth referrals. We will explore how to give our patients an experience that is so rare in our industry, people will beat down our doors, accept limited hours, and pay more money for it.

Don't get me wrong; I understand that everyone has different definitions of what success is. This book is not about how much more money you can take home every year, though that will be the result if you employ these principles. More money by itself is generally unfulfilling. What's important is to recognize that if we can take home more money per hour while we are at work, we then have the freedom to choose what do to with the extra cash flow and extra time we've created. We can work less hours, take on an associate, give more to the team, give more to charity, take more vacations, or be more involved in our communities. And yes, we can even buy a shiny new car or that boat we've been dreaming of. If we have great patient flow and a great patient base, we then have the freedom to have less accommodating hours, pull out of lower-paying insurance plans, or have stricter payment policies. The possibilities are endless when you're a heroic dentist who's leveled up his dental practice.

We have the best profession in the world. It's time that we capitalize on that fact and allow it to give us the best life possible. Dr. David Maloley says that an epic life starts with an epic practice. Are you ready to leap obstacles and win your way through to the epic practice? The time is now.

Homework

How does your practice stack up? What should your goals be if you want to become even better than average? It's time to take stock of your practice.

Get your most important facts and figures down on paper. Write down what they are now, and what you wish they were. What is your hourly, daily, weekly, monthly, and annual production? What percentage of your staff turns over each year? How many new patients do you get a month? What percentage of them are from external marketing? What percentage come from in-house referrals?

You may have other stats you enjoy tracking. This is the place to write them down, and write down your goals for them. Later in the book, I'll introduce you to the systems that will help you reach these goals, but until you choose your destination, you can't begin your journey.

CHAPTER 2
THE CALL TO AN EPIC FUTURE

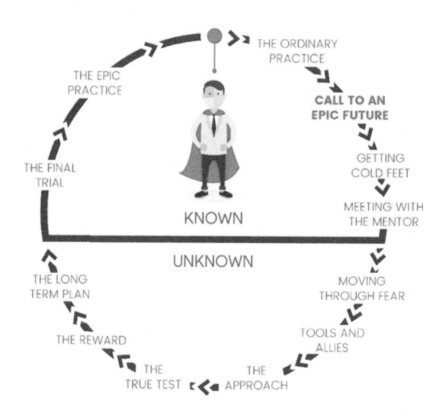

How can you make dentistry fun again? How can you challenge yourself, overcome obstacles, and save your practices from the forces of growing insurance networks and corporate dentistry? I'm going to give you some general principles to improve your practice and then do a walkthrough of the whole adventure for you.

Never forget that you are in control of your own destiny. There is more than enough dentistry to be performed in our country. There is no shortage of patients. I remember speaking to a dentist in his late 50's at a conference. He worked six days a week at two different practices because he needed to catch up on his retirement savings. He said that the insurance game had ruined dentistry and that his area was so oversaturated with dentists he couldn't fill his schedule.

I understood why he was upset, but it bothered me. Never play the victim. You have the resources; you just need to learn how to use them.

I asked this dentist where he practiced. He told me what town he practiced in. I asked how many dentists there were. He told me his estimate, hoping I would agree that his area was oversaturated. I asked him, "Is every practice in your town having the problems as yours?" He told me that they were.

I don't believe him. Somewhere in that town there is a dentist killing it. I know it because I am friends with that very dentist and his practice is remarkably busy.

Choose Your Own Adventure

We dentists rarely accept that where we are is a product of the decisions we've made. Let's get real. Let's take our success in our own hands.

Dentistry is a solved game, even though its solution wasn't taught in dental school. You can win it. You just need to learn the steps that will take you from where you are to where you ought to be.

At the end of the day, there are two major areas that comprise our net take-home pay: collections and expenses. You can increase your net income by either increasing collections or decreasing your expenses. The best way to increase your collections as a whole is to increase your production and then collect on that production.

There is a saying, "Don't step over dollars to pick up dimes." For the purposes of this book, we will be focusing on increasing production and collections, not decreasing expenses. Your expenses as a percentage of your total collections will largely decrease, but you won't be wasting time shopping around for cheaper supplies, labs, etc.

In my experience, most dental practices have a production and collection problem, not a spending problem. Once you have your practice cranking on all gears, you will then be able to "pick up those dimes", because you will have already "picked up all the dollars."

This is not a book about running multiple practices, though the principles will help you run any number of practices. This is a book about overcoming obstacles and meeting goals at work so that your life becomes fun again. It's about giving you the freedom to do the things you really enjoy. It's about being a hero in your chosen life, and facing obstacles head-on and with a positive outlook.

To face those obstacles, you need three things: a commitment to leadership, a great team to back you up, and systems that get you to where you need to be.

These three work together in what I call the *circle of dental prosperity*.

THE CIRCLE OF DENTAL PROSPERITY

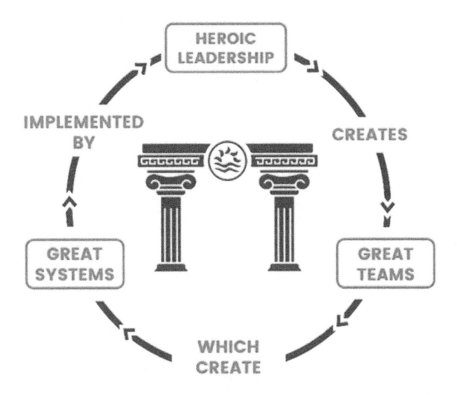

HEROIC LEADERSHIP

IMPLEMENTED BY

CREATES

GREAT SYSTEMS

GREAT TEAMS

WHICH CREATE

Heroic leadership creates great teams. Great teams create great systems which are implemented by leadership and great teams creating greater systems which are implemented by… LEADERSHIP…and so on and so on. Just like Odysseus conquered successively harder challenges and monsters until he could take back his kingdom, this circle lets you 'level-up' your practice and tackle ever more challenging goals.

A very important concept to understand is that heroic leadership bridges the gap between ideas and implementation. Without leadership, nothing is accomplished. Without leadership, everything falls apart. In the next chapters I will talk about leadership, great teams, and great systems; but first you must know what you want your practice to look like.

As Stephen Covey writes in *The 7 Habits of Highly Effective People*, "Begin with the end in mind."

A Practice Fit for a Hero

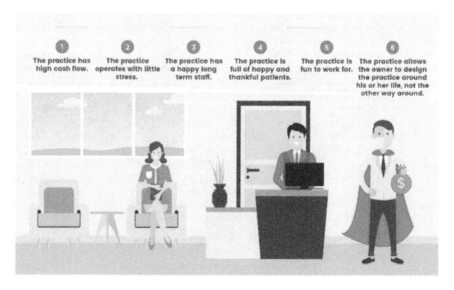

①	②	③	④	⑤	⑥
The practice has high cash flow.	The practice operates with little stress.	The practice has a happy long term staff.	The practice is full of happy and thankful patients.	The practice is fun to work for.	The practice allows the owner to design his or her life, not the other way around.

What makes a practice great? In my opinion, these are the six marks of a dream practice.

1. **The practice has high cash flow.**
2. **The practice operates with little stress.**
3. **The practice has a happy long term staff.**
4. **The practice is full of happy and thankful patients.**
5. **The practice is fun to work at.**
6. **The practice lets the owner design the practice around his or her life, not the other way around.**

When you find a real-world practice with these traits, it's about as close to a perfect practice as you can get.

1. The Practice Has High Cash Flow

When cash flow is good, everything else is good. If you go an entire day without seeing a new patient, but cash flow is good, life is still good. If you get sick and have to cancel an entire day of great production, but cash flow is good, you can rest in your bed without feeling like you should have just "sucked it up" and gone to work. If you need to replace a broken piece of equipment and cash flow is good, no big deal. A dream practice always has great cash flow. It's a must. We will build on how later.

The main idea here is that when cash flow is good everything else has the chance to be good as well.

Stress is lower, the doctor is happier and more comfortable, and the staff can work with someone who is pleasant to be around instead of a stressed out grump who is desperate for a dollar so payroll can be made. Treatment acceptance is better because the staff doesn't seem desperate to make a sale. That leads to more production and even better cash flow.

2. The Practice Operates with Little Stress

A lack of stress at work is key for a dream practice. You need to make your practice as stress-free as possible. You will spend a considerable portion of your waking hours at work. Why wouldn't you want it to be low stress? Stress is a mood killer. Stress makes everyone miserable. Have you ever seen someone act very unkindly, and when they finally apologize, they say, "I'm sorry, I'm just really stressed,"?

Stress is a nasty beast!

My most common stressor is overbooking. When my practice is overbooked, the patients don't get sat on time, I don't spend enough time building relationships with my patients, and then staff and I run around in an eight hour long fight-or-flight episode. These are not fun days and the patients can sense it. We want to work in a relaxed environment that is fun.

Nobody wins when we are stressed.

3. The Practice Has a Happy Long Term Staff

Think about what it is like to train new hires at your practice. It takes time. If you can retain staff, you rarely have to train new people. We should strive to have as little staff turnover as possible.

How much time do you spend at your practice? It's a lot of time to be spending with the same people each day. You need to love and appreciate your staff and you must be genuine about it. Work is more fun when you have great people to enjoy it with. If a staff member is toxic, get rid of them. Set high but realistic standards for your staff and hold them to it.

If you ask most people why they work, they will say for the money. I will tell you it's not. The largest reason people go to work is to feel appreciated and valued. That's it! I mean it. Smaller reasons are to work together for a common goal and for the relationships workers have with their coworkers. By and large though, it's to be appreciated. A happy staff begins with a heroic dentist who is grateful for their help.

4. The Practice is Fun to Work At

Most dentists spend four days a week seeing patients. That doesn't include the time to pay the bills, run reports, and run the business. Let's say the average dentist spends four 8-hour days seeing patients, and then another three hours running the business and other things. That means around a third of our waking lives are spent being a dentist. When we bring work stresses home with us, it feels like even more.

Based on the amount of time we will spend working, we should enjoy what we do. We should have fun every day. We need to create a great environment for ourselves and our teams.

This—creating a stress-free, fun practice—is one of the hardest 'monsters' you'll have to face as a dental hero. But if you can pull it off, you'll reap the rewards for the rest of your working life.

5. The Practice is Full of Happy and Thankful Patients

Your practice would be perfect if only you had perfect patients, right? Well, if you're a dental practice hero, you can create the perfect patients—patients who love you, appreciate what you do, and who swear you're the best dentist in town. The key is having a systematic way of creating a great patient experience. When you take great care of people enthusiastically and genuinely, your patients will be thankful. They will wait months to see you, they will adjust their schedules to be seen by you, and most of all, they will be thankful for the service you provide.

At my practice, our patients love us! Did I mention already

that it feels good to be appreciated? At some point, raving fans will be all the marketing you need to thrive and, guess what? Patients that come in from a word-of-mouth referral are the best there are.

6. The Practice Lets the Owner Design Systems around His or Her Own Life

Do low new patient numbers force you to work Saturdays? Are you forced to work late hours that you don't enjoy? Do you feel guilty about taking vacations? If you answered yes, then stop it!

We work so that we can live our lives. Our lives cannot be all about work. We need time to de-stress and spend time doing the other things we love. Do you have hobbies? Do you have some things you wish you had more time for? We all do.

The journey you're about to take will give you freedom.

If every cylinder of the practice is firing and we have lots of patients that want to see us, as well as many recall patients that still love to see us, we then have the freedom to lessen our insurance participation, have better hours, have stricter scheduling policies, and take more vacations.

Everyone loves a hero, and by taking this journey, you'll become that heroic dentist who patients love. What's important is that you determine how you want to live, and then make the practice work within those boundaries.

Don't wait for someday to enjoy your life when you retire. Enjoy it now. If your only goal is to bust your butt each week to sock away tons of money so that you can retire early, then you are probably so ambitious that you will be bored out of your mind once you do retire.

Our children are only young once; don't miss it for that magical "someday" when you can start enjoying life. Life will have already passed you by.

We have such a great profession that as dental practice owners we are allowed the flexibility and earning potential to really have a fantastic and rewarding life. Get out there and go get it!

Homework

Does your practice meet the definition of a successful practice? Turn to a fresh page in your notebook and list the six marks from above: Cash Flow, Low Stress, Happy Staff, Fun Place to Work, Happy Patients, and Life-Work Balance. Rate yourself on a scale of one to ten for each item. Unsure where you fall? Write down a plan to find out.

Then pick your worst area, and circle it. As you read, see how you can apply what you're learning to making a concrete improvement in that specific area.

CHAPTER 3
GETTING COLD FEET

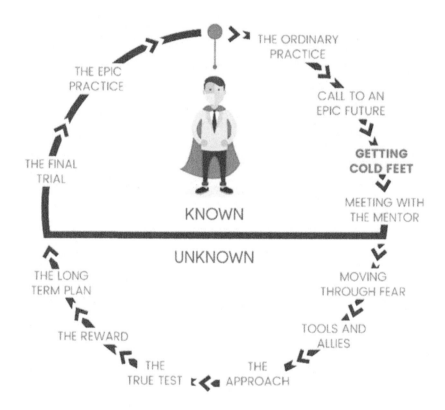

THE ORDINARY PRACTICE

THE EPIC PRACTICE

CALL TO AN EPIC FUTURE

GETTING COLD FEET

THE FINAL TRIAL

KNOWN

MEETING WITH THE MENTOR

UNKNOWN

THE LONG TERM PLAN

MOVING THROUGH FEAR

THE REWARD

TOOLS AND ALLIES

THE TRUE TEST

THE APPROACH

If you're like most people, you're probably a bit nervous about moving ahead at this point. You may think the dream practice I just described isn't possible. I assure you it is! Hesitation is normal for a hero. Before you set out on your quest, it's easy to focus on the roadblocks and obstacles in your way. The odds look insurmountable, especially if you have to go it alone. Risks seem foolish. After all, if you don't know anyone who's succeeded, doesn't that mean that failure is inevitable?

You may not feel like a hero to your team, your patients, and your practice. You know things are going wrong, but you're not sure where to start.

While every dentist is unique, every dentist's problems are not. Your main issues probably fall under a few big categories. You'll need to address them along your journey. So, what's holding you back?

The Broken Machine 13

In movies, there are usually a few pain points, places where the hero makes a big mistake and nearly dies. For instance, think of Cloud City in *The Empire Strikes Back*, or the snake pits in various Indiana Jones movies. Most dentists, like other heroes, tend to get tripped up by certain challenges. Let's look at the most common reasons dentists fail their practices.

Challenge #1: Lack of Positive Patient Experience

Why are you in the dental business? If you're having a great day, you might say, "To create perfect smiles." On a lousy day, you might answer, "To make money so I can retire to Aruba." Neither of these answers, however, is exactly right. You are in business to serve your patients. This means getting them healthy, but it also means giving them the sort of great patient experience that keeps them coming back to your office.

If you deliver a lousy experience, your patients won't come back. In fact, they might not go to any dentist. You'll have done them, and their teeth, a grave injury.

Meanwhile, if you consistently deliver great experiences, many of your other challenges disappear. What experience are you giving your patients right now? What experience do you wish you were giving them? We will go into depth on this later.

Challenge #2: Lack of Leadership

Does your team do what you want them to, or are you constantly having to berate them, correct them, and redirect them? A chaotic office comes from a lack of leadership. Your people want to do a good job. If you give them a strong example and a clear direction, they will meet and exceed your expectations.

It's not enough to have ideas and goals for the practice. A heroic leader communicates those goals clearly so that every single team member understands the philosophy and direction of the practice. If your office isn't what you want it to be, the first person to change is yourself.

Challenge #3: Lack of Systems

So, you have goals for the practice. How are you going to reach those goals? Without clearly outlined systems, you won't have a way to bring order to the chaos of your practice and create something amazing.

Systems are important because they develop into routines. They keep the practice running smoothly even when everything is busy. They let you deal with the current patient numbers and grow to become more productive. They free up brain power so that instead of making a million little, pointless decisions every day, you and your team can focus on the big things and deliver excellent care to every patient who walks through your door.

Challenge #4: Lack of Continuing Education

Dental school does a great job of teaching clinical skills. And our field has plenty of opportunities for continuing education if you want to perfect your skills or learn a new procedure. You can even schedule them to coincide with a family vacation to Hawaii or the Bahamas. There's no excuse to lack knowledge.

Many of us take the bare minimum requirement when it comes to CE. We never hear new ideas or learn new techniques to make us more efficient or profitable. The information is out there; we just don't take the time to hear it.

Challenge #5: Unsupportive Staff

When you want to make changes in your practice, are your staff excited, or at least nervous but positive? Or do they undermine you at every turn, holding fast to systems that aren't working? To succeed, you need staff that will support you in your goals and vision for the practice. If your staff are unsupportive, you have two options: mass firings, or finding a way to win them over to your side. The latter is your best option, I assure you. Unsupportive staff is almost always the product of poor leadership.

Challenge #6: Lack of Time to Manage Your Practice

A practice is not like a clock that you can wind up and then ignore. It takes tinkering. You need a few hours every week to run reports, see what's working, and come up with ideas to test. If all your time is spent on patient care or dealing with crises, you have no time to run the practice.

Challenge #7: Lack of Cash Flow

Cash flow gives you the freedom to travel for continuing education, buy new equipment, hire new staff, or change up your service mix. When you have enough cash on hand, you can AB test marketing campaigns, treat your staff to show appreciation, and take a leading role in your community. Without cash flow, you're focused on the present and can't plan for the future.

Challenge #8: Lack of Patients

Lack of patients can cause lack of production, lack of collections, and lack of cash flow. If you don't have patients coming in, you'll be too stressed to adequately plan for the future of your practice, and your team will start losing respect for you and the office, as they perceive a constant failure to attract new patients.

When you don't have enough patients to keep your practice afloat, you're in panic mode all the time. A practice without patients is a dying practice. I want you to be the sort of dentist who doesn't have to spend a lot of time chasing after patients. That frees you up to build great relationships with the people in front of you, the people who will become your biggest fans and proclaim your deeds to all their friends.

Challenge #9: Lack of Energy

If your practice hasn't been doing well, you may feel like it's a slog. You drag yourself in every day because you need to pay off your loans, but you feel like you're serving time, not serving patients. When you lack the energy to engage with your practice, patients and staff fall under the same spell of hopelessness and fatigue. Heroes are energetic. There's a spring in their step. They bounce higher and fight harder the longer they're on the job. If you feel drained, washed up, and blah, your lack of energy is killing your practice.

Challenge #10: Interpersonal Drama and Gossip

Your practice should be a fun place to work, where you, your staff, and your patients are happy. Interpersonal drama destroys that happiness. A high-drama practice feels like a war zone. The staff members engaged in the drama try to pull others in, and even being close to the action leaves people feeling exhausted and in need of a recharge.

It only takes one or two high-drama people to destroy your practice. As a hero, you need to learn to deal with drama on your team. Heck, even Luke and Yoda disagreed on occasion. But before you can deal with drama, you need to recognize the extent of the problem.

Challenge #11: Ineffective Marketing

Marketing is one of the tools of a heroic dentist who transforms his practice. Unfortunately, for most dentists it's a worthless tool. Does your marketing work? How do you know? Are you attracting the sort of patients who can benefit from your unique blend of skills, or just a hodgepodge of whoever saw that billboard out by the outlet mall?

If you don't have data to back up the effectiveness of your marketing campaigns, they're probably ineffective. That's the harsh reality of 99% attempts at dental marketing.

Challenge #12: Poor Service Mix

This is another common pitfall, especially for general and family dentists. Are you a one-stop shop for your patients, or do you need to refer out to specialists all the time? Do you offer some services that no one ever needs or wants? Are you remembering to tell patients about your services so they can make informed decisions about current and future treatments?

Service mix is a key component of keeping your schedule filled. Without the right service mix you'll get bored, have lots of open time, and you'll miss out on valuable opportunities. Is your service mix what you'd like it to be?

Challenge #13: Poor Billing and Collection Procedures

It doesn't matter what your service mix is or how many patients you see; if your billing procedures aren't efficient, you'll never have high collections. Aim for billing that is relatively painless for you, your staff, and the patient. Are most people paying upfront or using autopay options for bigger expenses? Are your financing procedures easy to understand and efficient at collecting payment? Billing is such a huge part of dentistry. Even if you're not as fast or as skilled at it as your billing department, you need to at least understand what's going on.

A Bonus Challenge

So what's the final challenge you face? It depends on who you are. While the thirteen pitfalls I outlined are the most common, you may have your own, unique challenges. Maybe your office is built atop a graveyard and you have poltergeist issues. Maybe sentient mushrooms menace you as you walk down the hall. Whatever the issues, name them now. You can't become a hero until you know what's holding you back.

Homework

How does your practice deal with each of the challenges I've listed? Be honest with yourself. Can you think of any times you've failed in these areas? Jot down those occasions. We will work on giving you some ideas on the next actionable steps in the chapters that follow.

What are your top three challenges at the moment? Write them down, and commit to have a plan for addressing them by this time next month.

CHAPTER 4
MEETING WITH THE MENTOR

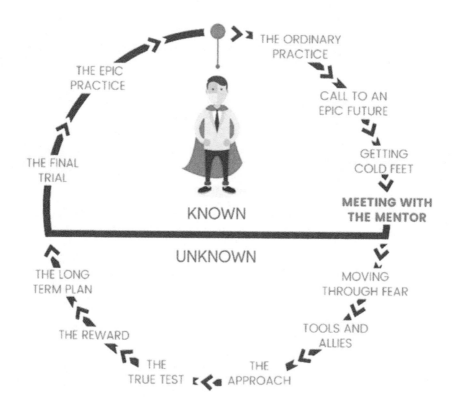

THE ORDINARY PRACTICE

THE EPIC PRACTICE

CALL TO AN EPIC FUTURE

GETTING COLD FEET

THE FINAL TRIAL

MEETING WITH THE MENTOR

KNOWN

UNKNOWN

THE LONG TERM PLAN

MOVING THROUGH FEAR

THE REWARD

TOOLS AND ALLIES

THE TRUE TEST

THE APPROACH

Every hero needs a mentor. Arthur had Merlin. Luke had Obi-Wan Kenobi. Link had that old man in the cave who appears, gives him a sword, and then never speaks again. You have me. I managed to go from dental school graduate to the owner of my dream practice in a relatively short time, and I want to help you enjoy what I have.

I graduated from University of Illinois School of Dentistry in 2009. I worked as an associate for two and half years at an office that was mostly managed care. I learned how to see high volume very quickly while working there. I also learned a lot of about what a dream practice is not. It's not that the office was an awful place to work, but it really lacked leadership, accountability, and efficient systems. The staff culture was indifferent at best, and the practice battled high turnover.

I decided to open a scratch start, near where I grew up, in 2012, just shy of the three year anniversary of my graduation. We grew very quickly. In our first full 12 months, we had $746K in collections. In our first full fiscal year we did $1.03M. Our second year was $1.36M. Our third year was $1.83M. Our fourth year was $2.15M. As I write, we are halfway through our fifth year and on track for $2.8M.

We're a five-chair practice taking PPO insurances with about 10 percent of our active patients FFS or cash. We have anywhere from 60 to 140 new patients a month. We had a two-year period where we stopped marketing completely because we couldn't see any more new patients. I added an associate in our fourth year and went down to seeing patients only three days per week. That freed up time for me to do other things, like writing this book.

You can replicate my success. At the end of your journey, you'll see a massive improvement in your production, collections, new patients, and most importantly, a large decrease in stress. Most of all, you will discover a new way of thinking about your practice that allows you to be the CEO of a business, rather than a technician in a tooth factory.

Homework

Think of your "dental story". Try to focus on how far you've come and the challenges you've conquered up to this point. Focus on those positives when you feel like you need some momentum for going forward. If you only focus on what you've done wrong, you're doomed.

CHAPTER 5
MOVING THROUGH FEAR

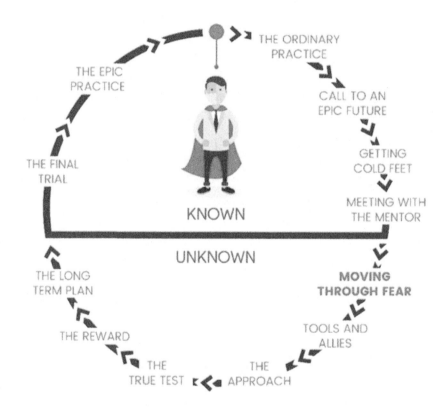

THE ORDINARY PRACTICE

THE EPIC PRACTICE

CALL TO AN EPIC FUTURE

THE FINAL TRIAL

GETTING COLD FEET

MEETING WITH THE MENTOR

KNOWN

UNKNOWN

THE LONG TERM PLAN

MOVING THROUGH FEAR

THE REWARD

TOOLS AND ALLIES

THE TRUE TEST

THE APPROACH

Adventures begin when the hero takes his first step outside his village and into the unknown. In that moment, he ceases to be a bit player and begins to be the leader of a team. Are you ready to become the hero of your practice?

A hero is someone who can transform ideas into actions and reach a goal. In popular culture, that's usually someone who sees a problem, comes up with a plan, and then recreates himself as someone fit to carry the plan out. If you take a look around your practice, there are probably areas where it's plagued by the forces of uncertainty, inattentiveness, or even chaos. It is up to you to fight through levels of inefficiency so that you can reap the rewards of a better practice.

When we were in dental school, we were (incorrectly) lead to believe that if we really focused on getting the clinical part of dentistry down, we were bound to be successful in our practice lives. Once we got into practice, it became very obvious that patients care very little about how excellent our dentistry is.

We can and should strive for excellence. Just keep in mind that your patients know almost nothing about the technical side of dentistry. They can be happy as a clam under the care of a bad practitioner for long periods of time, as long as they feel that they are heard, understood, and cared for.

To run a heroic practice, you need a different skill set. You need to focus on soft skills. Anytime we see practices "crushing it," we see leaders who give their practices a clear sense of direction, earn the respect of their teams, and repay that respect with obvious appreciation. If you fail to lead your team, you will spend most of your days micromanaging.

If you're not a leader, you have to do everything yourself. It feels like you're dragging the team up the mountain. The bigger your team, the more difficult it is to drag them up. In a good practice, the team charges up the mountain after you, ready to follow your lead because you've given them a clear direction and a shining example.

It's essential that you understand the fundamental role of you as the owner. You are the foundation of the practice. You show the staff what matters. They take their cues from you. Nothing that matters to the staff is going to get that way without first and foremost mattering to you. You're not just a doctor, you're in charge of a sales team. When I talk about sales, I mean ethical sales. Ethical sales means helping people see the value in what you offer and hence, converting them to happy buyers.

Your practice, whether you like it or not, at its very fundamental core, is a business. If you are uncomfortable about running your dental practice as a business and just want to do dentistry, then just keep doing what you are doing. Stay in your village. Refuse the old man when he offers you a sword. Let the lizard capture the princess.

But if you want to level-up your practice and win a great work -life balance, start thinking about your practice in terms of a business, and think of yourself as a business leader.

If you want your staff to be honest, take pride in their work, and connect with their patients, you need to be a leader who is honest, takes pride in your work, and connects with patients. If you do, your staff will follow suit. The staff needs a hero, and that hero is you!

This chapter is about being a leader in your practice. You need to set the example for what is acceptable and what is not. Then you have to inspire your staff to follow that vision. You will need to teach them, culture them, and motivate them to make your practice great. Like I said before, if it isn't important to you, it won't be important to them.

Just like a hero protects his companions from injury, you need to be the light that keeps the darkness out of your practice. The pastor at my church had a sermon discussing the fact that darkness is really just the absence of light. If you become the light at the practice, darkness will not overcome you. Be the hero, be the light!

Heroes Take Responsibility

I don't have enough fingers or toes to count the number of times I have heard dentists say they could do so much better if they only had better staff members. I've been at seminars where dentists have complained to each other about their teams almost as if it were some ritual. The problem with that sort of thinking is that, first of all, it makes you the victim and places your failures outside of your control. If you are one of those dentists that feel your team is holding you back, it is more likely that it is you holding back your team.

Jocko Willink, an ex-navy seal turned business consultant, discusses this in his book Extreme Ownership. He says, "the most fundamental and important truths at the heart of extreme ownership: There are no bad teams, only bad leaders." It's time to look at the man (or the woman) in the mirror. He goes on to say:

"In any team, in any organization, all responsibility for success and failure rests with the leader. The leader must own everything in his or her world. There is no one else to blame. The leader must acknowledge mistakes and admit failure, take ownership of them, and develop a plan to win."

For example, if you are overbooking, it's not the fault of your front office team. It's your fault by not being clear on how you want to be scheduled, not giving the team the training they need, or in the worst case, having the wrong people performing the task. When we begin to look at all the shortcomings in our practices as problems that we have created as leaders, we can then move forward to solve those problems. However, when we don't accept responsibility and become the victim, we become powerless.

Once you make the commitment to extreme ownership, you will begin to see everything through the lens of the leader. Only then can you begin to be the hero that your staff needs you to be. It all starts with you.

Wax On, Wax Off

There is no excuse not to practice, train, and grow your skills as a dentist and a leader. There are so many books, YouTube channels, podcasts, weekend seminars, online webinars, and mentorship programs that can help us become the leaders and clinicians our practices need us to be.

Successful dentists read constantly. Shut that TV off at night and start reading. I like to think that whenever I read a book, the way I look at the world has forever changed. Reading and a dedication to learning helped me build the practice I have today.

James Altucher, an entrepreneur who has founded or cofounded more than 20 companies says that "ideas have sex just like people do." They mate and have "idea children." The more ideas you have bopping around your brain, the more they'll pair up and produce totally new insights. If you don't add new ideas to the mix, your insights will start to look, for lack of a better word, inbred. You need fresh information and new experiences if you want to produce new insights.

So, where should you start looking for new ideas for your practice? Leadership and business books. It's good to read dental practice management books like this one, but branch out a bit. After all, you're leading a business. Let all those leadership and business ideas get cozy with all your dental ideas and create dental leadership babies. And don't just stop with books. Dental practice management podcasts and seminars can be even more valuable, because you get a chance to hear from multiple experts and to see what happens when they collaborate and connect.

Heroic Visions

You need a vision for your practice. Like Stephen Covey's, "Begin with the end in mind," we need to first know where we are going if we are going to get there. Defining your vision is pretty easy. Our vision at our practice is that we are going to give the patients such an unexpected and positive experience, that they will be happy to refer their friends and family. I have a lot of other sub-visions. For instance, "We are going to produce high quality dentistry and stand behind our work." Figure out what you want your practice to stand for. Make that your vision.

Along with vision, we also need goals. The goals have to be bigger than money. While production and collection goals are paramount for a great practice, the best goals are more personal. I have the goal that our practice runs smoothly each day, that no one is stressed out, that we enjoy the entire day, and that the patients enjoy it as well. There are a lot of smaller goals within that goal, but it's a great thing to strive for.

Write your personal and professional goals down. Once you have a goal, you can figure out the next actionable step and write that down too. Written steps help you progress toward your goals. As explained earlier in the book, the physical act of writing a goal down imprints it on your mind and commits you to it. Writing down a concrete, next actionable step will keep you moving toward your goals. So many of us freeze when faced with a huge problem. We fall into inaction because we don't know what to tackle first. "Next actionable steps" focus the mind and give you momentum and direction toward meeting your goals.

Set aside an hour one week and decide what you really want out of your practice and your personal life. Then track backwards and write all the little things that need to happen for your big goal to be completed.

No goal is too big, but every goal requires baby steps. For instance, if you want to lose weight, you know you could start by going to the gym, preparing your meals ahead of time, drinking more water, not eating past a certain hour, etc. But if you change too much at once, you'll fail.

Start with small things. Give your goals time to materialize after the summation of all the small goals you accomplish. It's really just about breaking your goals down into bite size pieces. Tony Robbins says, "We underestimate what we can do in a year, and overestimate what we can do in a month."

Ready, Fire, Aim!

Have you ever heard someone say they are going to start losing weight and be healthy, but that first they have to research some new diet technique or fasting regimen? We as humans like to convince ourselves that we don't know enough about something or don't have enough information to take action. But sometimes information gathering becomes a form of procrastination. You will never have perfect information. You need to go ahead and act.

I love the idea of "Ready, Fire, Aim" as opposed to "Ready, Aim, Fire". We need momentum, we need to move, and we can't fall victim to analysis paralysis. You will never know what is going to happen if you implement something new in your life. You can never foresee all of the possible outcomes before acting and no new changes will ever be perfect. If a ship isn't already in motion, the rudder can't steer it. So shoot first, then correct your aim to improve your results.

For example, I wanted to have my practice open from 7AM to 8PM four nights a week. I started with that goal, and then worked backwards through all the additional team members I would need, how we would schedule our five operatories, who would work when, when we would clean and maintain our equipment, etc. We tried to think of everything.

When we finally switched to split day and night shifts, it was chaotic. But we were able to make adjustments and address all the new issues that appeared. *Ready, Fire, Aim!* We got ready by making a plan, we fired by implementing, and we aimed by making adjustments.

One of my favorite quotes of all time comes from author Ray Bradbury. "Sometimes you just have to jump off the cliff and build your wings on the way down." After writing your goals and formulating a plan, take that leap; you'll figure out all the details on your way.

Be the Hero

Your leadership skills can take your practice to levels you never dreamed of, but your lack of leadership skills will always—and I mean ALWAYS—be the Achilles' heel. Leadership is everything!

It starts at the top. Strong teams never have weak leaders. Own everything that happens at your practice, especially the bad. Define your vision and goals, and then implement. Don't be afraid to get knocked down. Even though you are the leader and hero of the practice, you are going to get knocked down from time to time. That's OK; just jump up and keep trying.

Write down what your goals are for the practice and your personal life. Then work backwards and break them down into small actionable steps. You have to write these down! I'm going to say it again; don't just think about them! Get out that paper and start writing.

Better to Be Loved Than Feared

Every single interaction you have in the practice with a patient should be positive. So should every interaction with your team. We want to be likeable. Actually, we really want to be loveable. Think about the people you do business with. Why do you choose to do business with them? Chances are you like them. What about your best friend? I bet you find them pretty likeable.

When it comes down to it, it's not very hard to be likeable. It can be learned. There are tons of books on this subject. Dale Carnegie's *How to Win Friends and Influence People* is a great place to start.

Likeable people usually score high in most of these areas:

- Positivity
- Listening skills
- Being non-judgmental
- Empathy
- Authenticity
- Integrity
- Confidence
- Passion for their work
- Humor
- Willingness to touch
- Reliability
- Caring for others

Being liked by our patients is critical to treatment acceptance. Being liked by our teams is critical to the success of the practice. I had a mentor of mine tell me, "The key to being successful as a dentist is sincerity; once you figure out how to fake it, you are golden!" He was joking, but he had a point. If you can fake sincerity, or better yet, be sincere, patients and team alike will like and trust you.

Let's look at each of these areas in detail.

1. Be Positive

An optimistic, enthusiastic, positive outlook is infectious. Most of your patients don't want to be at the dentist. They're in pain, afraid, and mired in the present. Heroes, on the other hand, have hope and point the way to a better future. When you're positive, you give your patients confidence that your treatments can improve their lives.

Smile when you walk in the room, and smile when you leave. Be excited to see your patients! Energy is contagious.

Exhibit positive body language. Don't cross your arms or slouch when you are talking to patients. Ask your team if you are doing anything that seems negative while you are interacting with patients. It's a lot easier for a bystander to critique your people skills. Start working on those things.

2. Be a Great Listener

Make eye-contact with your patients. Ask questions and let them talk. People love to talk, especially about themselves. I once met a girl who talked about herself to no end. She never asked me anything about myself. I spent over an hour just listening to her ramble on and on. I really didn't like this girl, but guess what? She told my friend that I was one of the most interesting people she had ever met. She didn't know anything about me. She never took the time to ask. I was just a good listener.

Let your patients speak. Don't finish their sentences. Instead, practice active listening. Say things to your patients like, "What I hear you saying is_____; is that right?"

People want to be heard and understood. Give yourself the time to listen attentively and be present in the moment while they are talking.

3. Be Non-Judgmental

I think one of the greatest life lessons you can learn is that not everyone is like you. Everyone was raised in a different environment and has different values.

Joel Osteen tells a story about when he heard someone cussing out a cashier at the store. He said it was very easy to judge that person as wrong, but when he thought about it, he really didn't know how they were raised or what life experiences that person had up to that point that resulted in his being so vocal about his anger. Joel said that, for all he knew, that person may have handled it very well compared to how Joel would have handled it had he been in that person's shoes his entire life. We need to give everyone the benefit of the doubt and accept them for who they are.

4. Show Empathy

Let your patients know that you understand how they feel. If a patient says their tooth hurts, say "Oh gosh, that must be tough, tooth pain is the worst!" If a patient is acting embarrassed about their mouth, say something like, "I can understand that you might be feeling embarrassed about your mouth; a lot of patients feel that way when they first come in. We see that all the time and I promise that you are in great hands."

Pretty much any time a patient expresses negative feelings, you should throw an empathy statement at them. This will make people feel heard and understood. Isn't that what we all want?

5. Be Genuine and Authentic

Don't be stiff, be yourself.

Likeable people come in all shapes and forms. Some are loud, some are quiet, and either is acceptable. What is important is that you aren't being fake. People will see through that in a heartbeat.

6. Be Honest and Have Integrity

Tell the truth. Tell your patients what you would do if you were them. Your patient wants you to lead them to a decision. They need to trust that the decision you make for them is in their best interests. Honesty is the foundation of trust. You need to be trusted.

You also need to tell your patients what to expect with the dentistry you provide. If you raise expectations too high by not being truthful, you will breach the patients' trust when the reality doesn't match the promises.

Always operate with integrity in all that you do.

One of my favorite proverbs is, "Whoever walks in integrity walks securely, but whoever takes crooked paths will be found out." (Proverbs 10:9, New International Version). If you always do the right thing, you never have anything to worry about. You are secure. Never be afraid to apologize. If you have wronged someone, patient or team member, make it right. Your team will never get behind your vision if you don't build it on a foundation of integrity.

7. Be Confident and Secure

Portray confidence in your speech and body language. Look people in the eye. I cannot stress this enough. You will never appear confident if you can't look people in the eye.

Shake hands like you mean it. Don't crush them, but absolutely don't give them a little fish hand to hold. Someone who is confident bestows trust. Confident people are comfortable in their own skin. Everyone has bouts of insecurity, but understand that when you are dealing with patient care, you need to be confident in what you do. This is all part of leading the patient to treatment acceptance.

8. Be Passionate

Passion is about enjoying what you are doing right now. I can't even express to you how passionate about dentistry I am. It comes naturally to me. I absolutely love it!

If you absolutely hate dentistry, it is very unlikely you will be able to portray passion in what you do. Doing 36 hours of CE every three years to renew your license is not passion. Get passionate about your work. When you can exhibit passion to your patient about what you do, they will appreciate your enthusiasm and knowledge and will buy into your recommendations.

9. Be Humorous

Stop being such a stiff. Let loose and laugh. Never be afraid to laugh at yourself. Life is an awesome adventure! Lighten the mood a little.

10. Be Willing to Touch People

Shake people's hands, pat them on the shoulder, give them a hug! Dentistry is a very personal event for the patients. A simple touch demonstrates to the patient that you care about how they feel.

11. Be Consistent, Reliable, and Available

People love consistency. Think of a person who is in a different mood every time you talk to them. How much do you like that person?

Our practices need to be consistent too. The patient needs to know that the experience they got from us last time will happen again next time. That's what brand loyalty is all about: consistent delivery of consumer expectations that generate repeat purchases.

You also need to be reliable. Patients need to know that they can count on you. This goes along with being available. I give my cell phone number out to all my patients. I want them to know that I am their dentist 24/7, not just when we are open. The people you serve have put you in the place you are today. Be available for them.

12. Be Caring

Let your patients know that you care about them. We are in the caring profession. See your patients as people, not just teeth. Get to know them and start caring.

13. Be Attractive

Let's face it, we can't control everything about the way we look; but we can be well groomed, dress well, and smile a lot. Being attractive has a lot more to do with how we act than how we look. Have you ever met someone that was really good looking but when you starting talking to them you didn't like them anymore? On the other side, have you ever met someone not so physically attractive but once you got to know them you were enthralled? Charisma can be learned.

People Like Likeability!

Likeability is a skill set. Start learning it. Allow your staff to critique the way you interact with patients. This may be a big blow to your ego, but you are trying to take better care of people, so don't lose sight of the bigger picture. Your team will find your vulnerability refreshing.

Consider setting up a staff training on likeability. You probably have made an effort to hire people who are warm, friendly, and likeable; but everyone has room to improve. When you focus on likeability, it becomes an important part of your brand and helps transform your practice into a great place for patients, staff, and you.

Homework

It's time to take a hard look at yourself, and your abilities as a leader. Rate yourself on your ability to take responsibility, to have and communicate a vision, and to set goals. Be honest.

Now, look at the principles of likeability. How likeable are you, really? Which three of the principles describe you the best? What three describe areas where you have room for improvement?

Write down one concrete step for improving in each of those areas. For instance, if you need to get better at showing empathy, try to use one extra empathetic statement with each patient. If your appearance is an issue, commit to buying three new shirts that fit well or trim those nose and ear hairs.

CHAPTER 6
TOOLS AND ALLIES

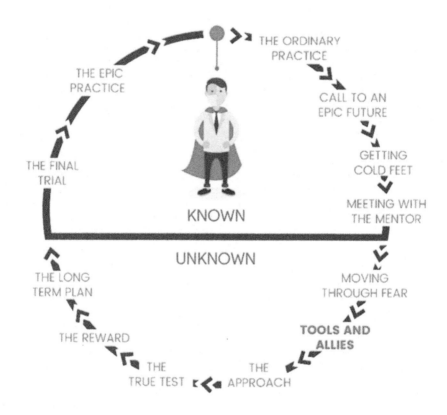

For heroes, no adventure can succeed without one or more sidekicks and a magical weapon of great renown. Your team are your comrades-in-arms, and your brand identity is the weapon that will propel you through challenges. It's time to prepare your team and hone your brand, so you'll be ready for the obstacles ahead.

The Hero Needs a Sidekick: Building the Dream Staff

You can't achieve a dream practice without a dream team. One of the core principles in James Collins's book *Good to Great* is to get the right people on the bus. A solid team is composed of many solid individuals. If you don't have the right people, you'll never get there.

Many doctors complain about their staff. They'll say, "If only I had more great people." I'm sure you already have a few stars on your team. You know who they are. You wish night and day that all of your staff could be that great. However, most doctors miss and gloss over the people in the middle who could become stars if they had the right training and environment. I'd go so far as to say that most of the people on your team have the potential; you just need to nurture it.

Have you stated your vision and communicated it to your team?

Start there. Define your brand and your expectations. Communicate them, then live them out. Lead by example. That's the easy way to develop the dream staff. It's all about extreme ownership. You have to walk the talk and lead.

Granted, you may have a few toxic individuals on your team. Ask each team member privately if there is anyone that is holding the team back in their opinion. You will see a pattern.

Don't let a bad apple keep you from your dream practice. These apples exist, but not to the extent that most doctors believe. Discuss your concerns and expectations nicely with them. If they refuse to change, let them go.

Hiring the All Stars

The problem with finding all-stars for your team is that they often aren't the ones looking for work. If they're already part of a great practice, they're not going to leave it for yours. In fact, these all-stars rarely even leave *bad* practices. Occasionally a great team member does become available, usually because they felt underappreciated at their previous job. These are the rare finds. More often, you will hire average people because, on average, people are just that—average.

The great news is that you can train about anyone, as long as they have the right attitude. I like to hire people who are outgoing, smiley, and fun to talk to. That's it! If you aren't those three things, you don't belong at my practice.

My interviews always consist of only talking and getting to know the candidate. The job applicant will always be on their very best behavior. They know how to answer the usual interview questions. Most people can put on a mask and say the right things if prompted. But if they can't be outgoing, smiley, and fun to talk to during an interview, chances are they won't be for the patients either.

I have always gone with my gut in hiring and have hired what I consider the absolute best team that ever existed. I don't have one person on my team whom I have ever regretted hiring.

At the time of this writing, my office has 17 employees. We haven't lost a single employee since we opened, except for those moving away or going off to college. Hire for the attitude, train for the skills, and you'll have a team worthy of a hero.

To train your team and onboard new employees, focus on the importance of your practice brand and culture. It's easy and fun to join a practice where everyone is moving in a positive direction cohesively as a team. Where does that positive direction come from? It comes from you. When you're clear about the brand and the expectations for the practice, the team knows which way you want them to go.

Culture is Everything

I remember my first associateship out of dental school. It was poorly managed. There were rarely meetings and patient care was very poor. They hired a new assistant. On her first day, she said to the other assistants in the sterile area, "I can't believe how big and busy this place is; it's awesome!" To which one of the other assistants replied, "Just wait two weeks, honey. You'll see what a shit hole this place is!" The other assistants nodded and laughed.

What do you think that new hire thought about her new job then? How long do you think it took until she believed what she was just told? Probably not long.

How does your staff feel about your practice? Wouldn't it be awesome if they would tell the new hire, "This is the best place I've ever worked!" It happens at my practice. It can happen at yours.

How do you know if the culture is bad at your practice? Just look at your turnover. Are people leaving? That's a pretty good indicator. The knee jerk reaction for most dentists is that those were bad employees to begin with. If you have that thought, go back to the Extreme Ownership idea. Guess what? It's probably because of you. Any practice with high turnover has a poor leader at the helm. Own it! One of the top reasons that employees leave a company is because they do not like their immediate supervisor or their boss. If you want to keep the staff around, you have to start playing nice.

Fill Them Buckets!

When my oldest daughter was three, someone bought her a new book. It was called *How Full is Your Bucket? For Kids*, by Tom Rath and Mary Reckmeyer. It explains that everyone in the world has an invisible bucket over their head. When people make them feel good, their bucket fills, and when people make them feel bad, their bucket spills and empties a little. Felix, the main character, goes through the day seeing how events affect his bucket. Later he realizes that when he fills other people's buckets by helping or being nice, it also fills his own bucket.

Apply that simple principle to your staff. How full are their buckets? Are you an instrument thrower? Doctors like that really do exist. How full are the buckets of that doctor's staff? Probably running on empty. I assure you that doctor's bucket is probably poorly filled as well.

We want a practice where everyone's bucket is full so that we can fill the buckets of our patients. Thankful patients will fill the team's buckets to some extent, but you, as the leader of the practice, are the main bucket-filler for your team. The way you interact with your team and affect their buckets has a direct correlation with the culture of your practice and your bottom line.

Here are some easy ways to start filling the buckets of your team.

1. Appreciate Them!

Remember that average dentist salary? If you want to be more than average, you have to have great staff. You can't do it without them. Have you told your staff how much you appreciate them? A simple thank you at the end of the day is a good place to start. Gratitude goes a long way.

I often text my staff members at night to tell them that I'm really happy they are part of the team and that I really liked something they did that day. Now, you can't do it too much or it will lose its value; but make sure you thank and compliment them on specific acts. For instance, on my day off, I called the practice to see how it was going. One of my front desk girls answered the phone. She always sounds enthusiastic and very welcoming when she answers the phone. The first thing I said to her was, "Wow, you always sound so nice when you answer the phone! I'm so happy we have you at the practice!" I'm sure she felt good about that. Some water just went into her bucket!

Every year at our Christmas party, I give each team member a Christmas card in which I write a few paragraphs about how thankful I am to have them working for me and what they do that makes them special. I promise you this isn't hard to do, though it did take me quite a while last year as we were up to 16 employees. I want to emphasize that this is not fluffy BS. I really mean what I write.

I have had many of my employees text me at night to say they were thinking about the practice and that they have never in their life worked for someone so appreciative. They always get me a gift for boss's day and take the time to write thoughtful and nice things about working for me. It fills my bucket. Everyone can have a full bucket! And full buckets fill other buckets! Start thanking and complimenting your staff. It will make them happy to come into work each day, and it will make you happy to work with them.

2. Be Generous!

Pay your staff well; this will be easy once you start growing your production and collections. You can pay your staff well above average and keep your staff costs in line with the recommended 22-28% of monthly expenses. They are the most valuable capital you have at the practice.

Buy them things, take them places, and celebrate with them! If a staff member needs new tires and money is tight, buy her an $800 gift card to a tire place. If she talks about this new Shark vacuum she is thinking about, buy it on Amazon and have it shipped to her house. If she is going through a divorce and money is tight, give her a bonus to help. Take care of your people. And let's be honest, when cash flow is good, it's fun to give!

Don't let staff leave your practice over a raise. A dollar raise is a lot more cost effective than hiring and training a new team member. I like to pay my staff their base wages, and then a bonus of 15% on any production that is above whatever we would need to produce monthly to keep staff costs at 25%. This usually amounts to around another $3–6 an hour. It also guarantees that my staff costs won't get out of control relative to collections. Even more importantly, it allows us all to share in our success at the practice. Never forget that we are in this together!

3. Get Together and Be Friends!

You need the staff to spend time together outside of work. I am not saying that we get together every weekend, but it's important to have work functions that aren't in the practice. If the staff members get along and are close friends with one another, they will work together as a team and create a fun work environment. If your employees are having fun at work, they won't leave to work somewhere else for higher pay if that opportunity comes up.

Think of your closest friends. How did you get to know and like each other? Chances are that you spent a lot of time in close proximity to each other. We often become friends with people at work because we are always around them and they are familiar. Take it to the next level, and get together outside of work.

Send them on a spa day in a limo. Send them to a concert. Plan a ski weekend. Go to the NASCAR race and tailgate. Pay them to go if it is on a day they would normally be working. Take them out to dinner and have a meeting. Fly the whole team somewhere for some CE. Build your team. It is not going to build itself; you need to put in the time together, and the time isn't going to schedule itself. Just do it! There are so many fun things you can do with your staff.

4. Train Them and Put Them to Work

Your staff wants to play an integral part in the patient procedures. Invest in them. Find out everything they are allowed to do by law and let them do it. They will value their job much more highly if they can contribute more to the overall process of dentistry. And, even better, letting them do more frees you up for more production.

For example, after I prep a crown, I take the impression (scan) with CEREC and let my assistants design, mill, glaze, adjust, and prepare the crown for cementation. You might worry, "What if they blow out the interproximal contact?" They do sometimes, and they know when they do and that it isn't acceptable because I have trained them. Occasionally it happens, and then the assistant will bake more porcelain on and continue. I don't walk into the room until it's ready to cement. After it's cemented, I check the occlusion. It's perfect almost all of the time.

What about making temporaries? Some dentists will lose their mind over the thought of it. Do you really think you need post-graduate training to make a temporary?

You don't, plain and simple.

Train your assistants to make the temps. Work with them, evaluate them, and improve on their skills. The time savings you will get from training them will be exponential throughout your career. Still, the best part is that they will enjoy doing it and will feel more accomplished than an assistant that just "sucks spit" all day.

Can hygienists anesthetize in your state? If so, send them to a seminar and get them certified. I anesthetize around half of my patients each day. It allows us to help more people and gives me the chance to keep producing in another room.

Is your perio program bad? We know that around 30% of the hygienists' gross should be in perio. If perio is underdiagnosed, send your hygienists to a seminar to learn the overall effect of perio on the health and what a value they are providing by diagnosing and treating it. I rarely talk about perio with patients. My hygienists have already done it by the time I walk in the room. I just have to confirm and move on.

What about your front office staff? There are great resources for training them. Front Office Rocks and Allstar Dental Academy are two awesome resources for training your team members online.

Your team is the most valuable capital you have at the practice. You need to invest the time, money, and energy in them. Not only will they appreciate it, but your bottom line will see the difference!

5. Hold a No Agenda Meeting

I try to meet individually with each team member on a regular basis. I learn so much from these meetings. I always tell them that if they are unhappy about anything, I want to know about it so we can address it. I even ask them how I am doing as their boss. That's kind of scary for some people. Get out of your comfort zone and start communicating with your team. You'll be amazed at the valuable information that provides.

These meetings can only yield fruit when your staff knows that they can trust you, and that you won't gossip about what happens in the meetings. If they have reason to suspect that, for instance, when Susie complains about Ann, you'll tell Ann who complained, they won't trust you.

Your team has to work together every day, so if anyone thinks you'll use the information to turn people against each other, even inadvertently, they won't say anything at all.

As a doctor, you would never know much of what you hear in these meetings unless a team member brings them to your attention; so if you act on information immediately, people will know who "squealed".

Instead, use the information you get to find a way to personally observe problematic behavior. That way, when you call it out, the staff member will know the correction comes from you, not from one of their teammates.

6. Integrity is the Core Value

One of the things my father instilled in me was a great respect for integrity. Integrity is critical to being a leader.

This boils down to three things: You do what you say you will do, you do the right thing, and you do it for the right reasons.

Zig Ziglar—an author, salesman, and motivational speaker— once said, "It is true that integrity alone won't make you a leader, but without integrity you will never be one."

Your team needs to know that if you make any decision, that you are doing it for the right reasons. Leaders without integrity can't be trusted, and they can't build strong relationships with their teams.

If you don't have a strong relationship with your team, you can't begin the journey to a better practice.

A Culture of Coachability

Teach your staff that every failure is a learning experience. Every patient complaint is a blessing, because it gives you a blueprint for growth. Failures let you recalibrate. When staff no longer fears failure but are willing to learn from it, you've created a culture of coachability. You've created a space in which you can lead and inspire. Be an educator, not a criticizer. If you publicly criticize your staff members when they do something wrong, you'll never have a coachable team.

Give the staff permission to criticize you as well. My staff constantly tells me things I can improve on. I appreciate the fact that they trust me enough to tell me the truth and that they understand our shared goals for the practice. In fact, they understand our goals so well that they can see when I'm not meeting them!

Finally, if you lose your temper or hurt someone's feelings, step up and apologize. Let them see you accept your own failures, make reparations, and try to do better. No one wants a coach who seems less of an adult than they are themselves. Be the adult in the room. Mentor, don't hector, and you'll have staff who are eager to learn and improve.

Taking a (Heroic) Hit for the Team

As the leader of your team, all mistakes are ultimately your responsibility, and you need to take responsibility for mistakes. For instance, if a lab case didn't arrive and your assistant didn't bother to check until the patient was in the chair, go in there and apologize to the patient without blaming your assistant. Everything that happens under your roof is your problem. Nothing will build more loyalty than you being able to take a bullet for your staff. Do it.

Remember extreme ownership? You need to lead like a hero.

Staff are People Too!

A great practice is a lot like a marriage: it requires great communication! Never be afraid to be honest with your staff and they won't be afraid to be honest with you. Always have the attitude that you are available to address any concern they have.

Communicating the Numbers

Talk to your staff about the practice numbers. You don't need to share what you take home each year, but every member should know what the office produces and collects. They should know their reappointment rate and other key performance indicators that you feel are critical to the practice. They need to see how their individual numbers affect the overall profitability of the practice. Information helps them take pride in their performance and in the practice as a whole. Everyone on the staff should know their hourly production, the practice's collection percentage, and the new patient conversion rates. Teach them to run reports on these numbers, or post the numbers publicly.

Remember, numbers and goals help make work a game, and everyone wants to win!

One Bad Apple...

Sometimes at the office, it can feel like you are supervising a sandbox full of kids. Have you ever had a team member tell you something that someone else is doing that is bothering them? It can be how they answer the phone, or how they greet patients, or basically that they are not pulling their weight as a team member.

When someone on your team tells you something like this, the problem is often that they won't want you to address it with the other person, for fear that the person will know who tattled on them. I had this problem for a long time at my office, until we started doing what we call the "vote someone off the island surveys."

We used a free online survey website and created questions for each team member so that they could be rated by their peers. This survey needs to be short so it can be completed quickly, but more importantly, it needs to be anonymous. People in leadership positions would get a few more questions than other team members. For example, for me, my associate, and my office manager, we asked everyone the following questions, on a scale of strongly disagree to strongly agree.

Paul Etchison

	Strongly Disagree	Disagree	Neutral	Agree	Strongly Agree	Standard Deviation	Responses	Weighted Average
upholds the values of the practice.	0 (0%)	0 (0%)	0 (0%)	2 (12%)	15 (88%)	5.85	17	4.88 / 5
makes it clear the duties that are expected of me as a team member.	0 (0%)	0 (0%)	0 (0%)	1 (6%)	16 (94%)	6.31	17	4.94 / 5
provides guidance and direction to improve my skills and knowledge as a team member.	0 (0%)	0 (0%)	0 (0%)	3 (18%)	14 (82%)	5.43	17	4.82 / 5
values and appreciates me.	0 (0%)	0 (0%)	0 (0%)	5 (29%)	12 (71%)	4.72	17	4.71 / 5
gives me adequate praise when I deserve it.	0 (0%)	0 (0%)	2 (12%)	3 (18%)	12 (71%)	4.45	17	4.59 / 5
I feel comfortable discussing my concerns about the practice	0 (0%)	0 (0%)	2 (12%)	4 (24%)	11 (65%)	4.08	17	4.53 / 5
								4.75 / 5

All the other team members are rated on a scale of 1-10 on how well they uphold the values of the practice, and also how much they are a valuable and contributing team member. At the end of each team member's questions, there is a box where they can type praises or constructive criticisms.

What's absolutely wonderful about an anonymous survey is that it gives you the power as a leader to address issues without knowing who said what. It also allows everyone to praise and compliment each other.

Without surveys, you have all the children in the sandbox confidentially crying to you that Sally kicked sand in Molly's face, or took her toy shovel away, but not wanting you to say anything because they don't want to be the sandbox tattle tale.

The amount of information that I have received since beginning this has been amazing. Even better, it is more or less a performance review on everyone by their peers.

If you have a bad seed, it is going to come out. I think anyone scoring lower than an eight needs to have a meeting with you, so that you can address what issues they are having and what your expectations are. If they continually score low, you have to kick them off the island.

I also throw in some questions about the practice at the end of the survey as well. You can ask whatever you want to get some feedback on. It's great!

Bonus Systems

I strongly believe in bonus systems.

A search on DentalTown will yield many different options for team bonuses. I feel they are very motivating if you follow a few basic principles.

1. It Needs to be Immediate

Yearly bonuses don't do anything. I assure you that your team is not thinking about that final year end number in January. The same goes for monthly or quarterly bonuses. Long time frames won't get you real results. Base bonuses on daily or weekly goals, no longer than that.

2. It Needs to be Simple

Some bonus systems are so complicated that the team can't understand them. If they can't understand the rules, they can't play. Plain and simple. Don't over complicate things; it really isn't necessary.

3. Bonuses Need to be Cash-in-Hand

Bonuses should be paid out at the end of the day or at the end of the week. It's much more motivating when the team members leave each day with cash in hand for a job well done. These can be accounted for in your payroll as cash advances. Your team will have to pay taxes on this income. All you need to do is stop at the bank once per week and grab some cash so that you can pay these out.

4. Grab Sack Bonus

We used to do a grab sack bonus in which we had colored chips that were worth ten, twenty, or fifty dollars that the team would pick at the end of the day if we hit our production goal. If they hit it on Monday, they each picked one chip. If they hit it on Tuesday as well, they picked two chips. If they hit it on Wednesday as well as the two days before, they picked three and so on. You can do it any way you want. We did this for around two years until it started getting too complicated — once we picked up an associate and I had quite a few part-timers, who didn't work each day we were open. It was just getting too hard to get everyone together as our days ended at different times. Nevertheless, I really liked this system when we were smaller. It was tons of fun and it helped to bring the team together at the end of the day and talk about what worked and what didn't.

5. Weekly Bonus Based on Staff Expenses

This is our current bonus system. You take all your staff expenses for the month and divide by 4.33 to get your weekly staff expense. This includes payroll and any associated taxes, along with 401K contributions, and any other staff expenses like lunches or uniforms.

Now that you have what your staff costs per week, you need to figure out what you would need to produce that week in order to keep those costs at 25% of adjusted production. That is four times your weekly staff expense. That is your baseline weekly goal.

You can then take any amount produced higher than that and bonus a percentage of that to the team. I do 15%. You can divide it evenly or prorate it based on the amount of hours they work. I like this system because it guarantees that my staff expenses will never exceed 25%, and it allows us all to share in the profitability of the practice.

In my perfect practice model, everyone would be paid minimum wage and then would get a percentage of collections. That would be rather complicated, so this is as close to that as I can think of.

6. Specific Bonuses

You can also do specific bonuses on areas in your practice you want to improve. We did a monthly bonus if we got five online reviews for a while. On the other end of the spectrum, you can also take bonus money away if tasks like cleaning the lab or writing clinical notes are left undone.

You need to decide how you want to work it. Always make sure that the team understands that bonuses are just that, bonuses. They are not to be expected and they can change. They are rewards for performing beyond what is expected. If you set your goals too low and don't challenge the team, they will not be motivational anymore. Change your goals and bonuses accordingly.

You Need the Team

Without his team, a hero can't succeed. Never lose sight of all the things you are able to do because you have a great team. Occasionally, when things get really busy and your practice is firing on all cylinders, you will need to reground yourself and express your gratitude for how everyone at the practice made it all possible.

Be the boss that everyone dreams they could have. It isn't that hard. Be a good person, and appreciate every ounce of sweat your team puts in for you. If you are grateful and express that gratitude to the people who walk the trenches with you each day, you can never go wrong.

Branding is Not Just for Coca-Cola and Nike

If you're the hero of your dental practice and your team are your sidekicks, your brand is your secret weapon. A great brand helps you build a great practice. All of your competitors graduated dental school. Since they graduated, we assume that they can at least do bare minimum dentistry. Your brand is what lets you stand out from the crowd.

A marketing definition of a brand would be a unique identity, or a shorthand way the public thinks about what a business does, produces, serves, or sells; or the way in which they do it. So essentially, everything we do at the practice is branding. Brands help us to order different options in our minds. We think of specific things when we think about different brands. We obviously have different thoughts when we think about Mercedes vs. Kia when it comes to cars. We may have never had any first-hand experience with either of the brands, yet we have thoughts about what they mean and how they are different.

Brands are the identity the products and services have in the consumer's mind. They are fluid and always changing as well. If you grew up in the nineties, you will remember the Starter brand of jackets. They were what everyone wanted and people were willing to pay a premium for them. Now, twenty or so years later, Starter brand clothes are sold at Walmart. This changes the way the brand Starter is viewed. It is no longer a premium brand.

Brands also allow us to express ourselves, to show the world what we value and who we are. For instance, if you have friends who run, ask them about shoes. Some of them are Nike people, some are Asics people, some are Brooks people. It's rare to meet someone who switches brands of shoe. The shoes aren't just a tool to help them exercise while protecting their feet. They're part of who they are as a runner. People strongly identify with either Apple or Android phones as well. Have you ever gotten into an argument about which one is better? I'm sure we all have.

Brands and their identities help people make purchasing decisions as well. If you were on a road trip and had to use the washroom really badly, would you expect that McDonalds or Burger King has a cleaner bathroom? Most people would say McDonalds. Part of McDonalds' brand is having consistent standards for cleanliness at every location.

Brand images are created by advertising and marketing, as well as how the products or services deliver. I once read about a bank that did a study in which they had customers rate their customer service. They ran a TV campaign saying that they were a very personal bank and provided great customer service. At the end of the customer survey, they asked if the customer had seen any of their advertisements. What they found was that people who had seen the advertisements rated the customer service higher, and hence, had a more positive view of the brand over the people that had not.

Can we do this? Can we advertise that we are a great office that provides exceptional customer service? The answer is yes. We can put it on our website. We can put it on all of our print materials as well as our mailers. Mostly, our brand image will come from the way the patient experiences our practice when visiting or interacting with us over the phone. A great book is *Everything is Marketing* by Fred Joyal. One of the takeaways of the book is that everything we do in the office creates our brand. Everything from the way it looks, to the way it smells, to how we answer the phone—it all matters.

You may say, "I don't like all this fluffy marketing stuff!" That's fine. Guess who does like it? Corporate dentistry. You will get killed by them if you don't adopt this belief. Do you know who else likes branding their practice? The top one percent of dentists who are killing it week to week. Even if you think the whole idea is silly, I assure you that your office has a brand. If you don't think about how what you do in your office affects your brand, your brand probably stinks. Yet this is good news, because it is easy to differentiate your practice from the stinky ones just by looking around at your systems and making everything more customer service focused.

The Big Brands: What Makes Them Great?

If we start to think about the most powerful brands in the US, we will find something in common with them. A google search will tell you that they are brands like Coca-Cola, Nike, Apple, Microsoft, and Marlboro. Can you tell what they all have in common? They are *product brands*, meaning that they sell a product. Product brands are tightly managed through their advertising and packaging. They tell the consumer what to think about their brand. More importantly, it is very easy to be consistent and to deliver a consistent customer experience when the only way the consumer interacts with the brand is through advertising and buying their product.

If you want to introduce some inconsistency to a brand, add humans to it. Think about brands that require people to relate to humans when interacting with the brand. Those are *service brands*. Think of hotels, coffee shops, and airlines. When you rely on humans to deliver your brand message, you will always have some element of inconsistency. How many times has someone completely written off a company because of how they were treated by one employee? That employee could have just been having a really bad day, but the brand is forever tarnished in the mind of the consumer. When a brand gets a bad reputation, it sticks. It can make their attempts at marketing fall flat, or become bad jokes.

Every time a consumer interacts with a brand, it is called a *touch point*. Touch points can be on- or off-brand. What happens at each touch point either reinforces or ruins what the *brand promise* is. One thing to realize is that service brands have many more touch points than product brands. Every single touch point in our practices needs to be optimized so that it can reinforce our brand. We want to keep these touch points on-brand as often as possible. But, before we do that, we need to define our brand and what it means to be *on-brand* to begin with.

Think about BP's (British Petroleum) *brand promise*. I found this on their website:

"We help the world meet its growing need for heat, light and mobility. We strive to do that by producing energy that is affordable, secure and doesn't damage the environment. BP is progressive, responsible, innovative and performance driven."

So if that is their brand promise, do you believe it? What has your experience (or touch points) been with the company? I can tell you that after the gulf of Mexico oil spill in 2006, most people don't believe BP "produces energy that doesn't damage the environment," or that they are "responsible." What speaks louder, the promise or the experience? The oil spill was off-brand for BP, and most people would find their brand promise slightly hard to swallow after that disaster.

Brainstorm the attributes of your brand with your team. What is your *brand promise*? Decide what you want people to think about your office. Every touch point needs to be pleasant and reinforcing. They need to meet the expectations of the patient. When we are off-brand, we kill the brand and experience *brand erosion*.

I give new employees a brand manual. This is basically a manual that tells them that we all love what we do at the office and gives examples of the standards we set for the office. This is a great way to onboard new hires as it immediately sets the expectation that we are going to be very intentional about what experience we provide for our patients.

The Weight of On-Brand and Off-Brand Touches

In our practices, a patient moving from check in to check out can have an almost unlimited number of touch points. It only takes one to kill a case. Remember those balancing scales that we used in science class? You put calibrated weights on one end to balance the weight of the object you were trying to measure?

Case acceptance works a lot like that scale, with the one end being the patient saying yes, and the other tipping towards the patient saying no. The unfortunate part is the on-brand touch points weigh much less than off-brand touch points. Think of on-brand touch points as weighing one pound each. An off-brand touch point weighs fifty. That's why it's so critical to be consistent in what kind of service you deliver.

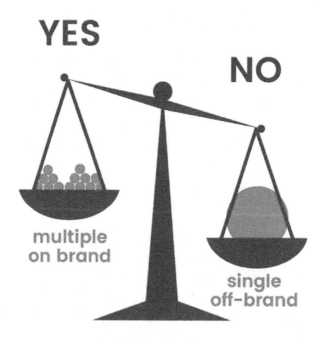

Branding at the Dental Office

We need a strategic and organized way to deliver *on-brand* customer experiences that magnify our *brand promises*. The way we provide customer service is how we put our brand in motion.

When we take customer service to the next level, we amplify our uniqueness and provide the patient with value that is much greater than expected. We totally exceed their expectations. If you do that in dentistry, you will blow your patients away, because again, it is so uncommon. Also, patient expectations at the dentist are so low to begin with, that it is unbelievably easy to exceed them if you focus on it, even just a little.

Patients want to feel trust. They need to feel that they aren't being cheated. They want us to have genuine concern for their problems and to appreciate them as people. They want to feel comfortable doing business with us.

These patient needs can help you begin to define your brand.

In my practice, my brand begins with a mission statement:

Our mission is to recruit the nicest, most generous, most honest, and authentic people we can find—who love dentistry and providing care to patients just for the fun of it and who see our business as an excuse to have a good time while providing a great service—and bring them together in a caring environment that provides our patients with the absolute most enjoyable dental experience possible.

That may be a little long, but I assure you if you come to my office, you will feel that vibe. Here are the brand promises that my staff and I came up with:

Hospitality – We take great care of people and mean it.
Amenities – Televisions on the ceiling, water bottles, coffee, warm towels after procedures, blankets, a spa like atmosphere.

Quality – We use the highest quality materials.

Efficiency – We are efficient, allowing our patients to have fewer visits and shorter time per visit.

On time – Our patients are seen promptly; our waiting lounge is for guests of patients, not patients themselves.

Warranty – We stand behind our work because we know it is solid.

Same day treatment – It's convenient for everyone.

Convenient hours – We are open until 8 pm four nights a week.

A single dental home – We have an extensive service mix, which minimizes our need to refer to specialists for the convenience of our patients.

High technology – We have CBCT, CEREC, digital x-rays, electric hand pieces, velscope, DIAGNOdent. Everything we have is state of the art, using all the technology available to dentistry.

Education – We take a lot of CE to stay current and knowledgeable on treatments and what is best for our patients.

Comprehensive treatment – We believe in treating the mouth as a whole, not tooth-by-tooth dentistry.

Relationships – We develop and maintain solid relationships with our patients.

Integrity, honesty, and authenticity – These are paramount to maintaining patients' trust and will not be sacrificed in anything we do.

Available – We answer our phones, we return phone calls, we give out the doctors' cell phone numbers for weekend emergencies.

Financing – We will be accurate in our treatment estimates and will honor them as agreements. We will find a way to work our dentistry into our patient's budget with financing.

A culture of coachability – We are always trying to improve the way we provide care. Everyone who works in the practice is free to constructively criticize each other when it comes to how we deliver our brand.

Friendly – We smile and touch the patients, we are excited to see them and they are our friends. We are enthusiastic.

If you don't define what your brand is, you can't define what actions are on- or off-brand.

Sit down with your team and create your own mission statement and brand promises. Feel free to steal mine. If you need more inspiration, *Branded Customer Service* by Janelle Barlow and Paul Stewart can help you get started.

If you define your brand, you can even handle complaints in an on-brand way. Let's face it, people are going to complain about something we did. But we can handle complaints in the right way by staying on-brand.

If you learn nothing else from reading this book, remember the idea of branding through service:

- Your office already has a brand, like it or not
- Every interaction with the patient is a touch point, and it establishes that brand in their minds
- To compete, you need to take control of your brand through every aspect of your practice
- You and your team need a clear sense of your brand identity
- Once you have articulated your brand with your team, you can see every touch point through the lens of on-brand and off-brand
- Try to eliminate off-brand interactions

When everything you do is on-brand, your patients will be ecstatic about the care they receive. If a patient experiences on-brand touch points from the moment they see your website all the way until they check out of their first visit, they will be completely overjoyed about the care they received and will be happy to tell their friends and family about it. They will be happy to publicly post a five-star review on google about you. They will also be happy to pay more for your services and accept that you have limited availability, since you are so popular.

Creating an On-Brand Environment

Patients are making judgements about you based on what they see and how they feel when they are in your building. Every chair, every wall, and every piece of art is a touchpoint for your brand. The good news is, unlike people, physical objects are easy to control and predict. Your physical environment is a great starting place for putting your brand identity to work.

Even better, it's not just your patients who observe and make unconscious decisions based on their surroundings. When your practice environment is on-brand, it's easier for your team to be on-brand too.

Take a look at your practice. A fun activity to do with your team is to play musical chairs. Everyone gets a pen and paper and sits in the waiting room, the bathroom, the sterile area, the hallway, the operatories, etc. Only one person per room. Then, sit and write everything you see. Write about the dirty ceiling, the old magazines, the scuffed up trim, the wall colors, the décor, etc. Write about everything. Every three minutes, switch. Once everyone has been in every room, bring all your papers to one meeting place and discuss what you see. This will be a good starting point to what you need to change, because if you see it, your patients do too.

Take a hard look (and listen and touch and smell) around your practice, to make sure that the physical environment supports your brand in the following areas.

1. Colors and Cohesiveness

Your color scheme should be consistent throughout the practice and on all your internet and print materials. Consistent colors help things flow and give patients a unified experience.

2. Uniforms

Staff uniforms should match to increase cohesiveness and team spirit. There's a reason that schools and sports teams show their spirit through shared colors. Update uniforms frequently to keep them from looking worn.

3. Doctor Attire

Never wear scrubs. Stick to business attire. It makes a big difference in how your patients see you. It's hard to close big cases in your pajamas.

4. Doctor Hygiene

You are your number one brand ambassador. If you look sloppy and unkempt, people will think your work is sloppy too. Keep your ear hair, eyebrows, and facial hair well-trimmed. Rinse with Listerine before consults, or chew some sugar-free gum to give yourself fresh breath. How many people have you heard say that their dentist had the worst breath they ever smelled? Don't be that guy or gal. Also, wash or pat your face before you talk to patients. We all know that moving from room to room while wearing business clothes can make you sweaty. Don't walk into that consultation looking like Patrick Ewing or Shaquille O'Neil during the fourth quarter of a basketball game; get yourself together.

5. Doctor and Staff Teeth

You wouldn't take weight loss advice from an obese person, so don't expect your patients to take dental advice from someone with bad teeth. Your entire staff should have straight and white teeth. If they do not, provide it to them at no cost. Either do it yourself or pay for it. That goes for you as well. Straighten out those lower incisors, because let's face it, crooked teeth do not look healthy. We are in the dental health business, so we need to have beautiful smiles.

6. Your Waiting Room

Your waiting room should be homey and relaxing. Your patients are already nervous and unhappy to be there. Give them surroundings that induce calm by making it look like a living room, not a clinic. Get rid of those tiny plastic clinic chairs. You know what I am talking about. You want to differentiate yourself from that. Go to Value city and buy some affordable but nice-looking chairs. You can replace them in four or five years when they are falling apart.

Instead of the brochures, mount two televisions in your waiting room—one that the patients can control to watch any television they choose, and the other that you will create a slide show to show pictures of the team, their families, and some before and after of your work or what services you offer. This accomplishes two things: It allows the patient to see you and your team as people who have families and also allows them to see what procedures you do that they might not know about. Put some pictures of team events you went to with your team. You want to give the vibe that everyone is personable and gets along with each other. Hopefully that's the truth!

Throw some slides in between that show a staff member smiling next to the text, "How can I help you?" Make some slides that say things like, "At our dental office, if we didn't provide you with the best dental experience you have ever had, then we have failed." Or try, "If there is anything we can do to make your visit more enjoyable, please don't hesitate to ask." Remember that bank study where people felt better about the customer service when they saw the advertisements? Use that to your advantage. The possibilities are endless.

Have bottled water and a Keurig available for patients to use. You would be blown away by how quickly patients go through the coffee at our practice. Does drinking coffee make you feel comfortable? I bet you do it at home when you are comfortable. Why not at the practice? This conveys a culture of taking care of people. It is our brand and we can express it by offering amenities to the patients. They will appreciate it, I promise.

Make a book of your clinical cases. Patients love to look at these. Just print pictures and put them in an album or do it in a binder. Leave that on your waiting room table. You can also print these into books online. You will also want to have magazines, as these are expected, but don't go overboard so that it becomes clutter and most definitely don't store these on the table. Place them on a wall hanger where they can be organized and look nice.

Play some spa music lightly in the waiting room. It will add a nice touch. Don't forget to burn some candles or get a scent machine. We use one from Scent Air. It is around $100 per month but is well worth it. Patients always comment on how good our office smells. Think of the difference in subconscious feeling that your patients will feel when smelling something nice as they walk into your office, as opposed to burnt teeth and formocresol.

It all adds up.

7. The Bathrooms

These should be the nicest rooms in your practice. Don't cut corners here. Get the marble, and buy a nice mirror. The bathroom must be exceptionally clean at all times. To your patients, a dirty bathroom means you use dirty instruments.

I like having the same spa music playing in the bathroom as I do in the waiting room. It's like a refuge that the patient can go into before their appointment. It's a really comfortable room. We also have Listerine and cups for rinsing, as everyone is always self-conscious about their breath when they are about to have someone fudging around in their mouth. Use a plug-in for smell in here.

We've hit on elements of sight, sound, taste, smell, but what about touch? DON'T BUY CHEAP TOILET PAPER!!! Just don't do it. All these things add up to a big effect.

8. The Front Desk

This area must be clean and organized. Buy some office organizers and get rid of the clutter.

I remember at my wife's and my fertility doctor's office: We were having a consult with the doctor and he had papers everywhere! I know we have all been there, but think of the impression it made. It just seemed like a big mess. I didn't really think anything much of it at the time, but as soon as they dropped the ball on an issue dealing with treatment, my mind immediately went back to that desk. I started saying to my wife, "No wonder they screwed that up; did you see the doctor's desk? It was an unorganized mess. That man pays no attention to detail. And their pictures in the waiting room are crooked. That office doesn't give a crap about anything other than taking our money!"

Your patients make the same sorts of judgements about you

based on your office. Stress to the team the importance of having everything tidy and organized, as it speaks to the quality of our dentistry and maintains the brand image.

9. The Hallways

These need to be clean and vacuumed often. Get the carpets cleaned or replaced regularly. Everything needs to look pristine as the patients travel through the office. Again, you want to set the example. If you walk by a paper point or burr sitting on the floor all day long without picking it up, don't expect your staff to bend down and pick it up. Do it yourself.Walk the walk and set the example.

10. Operatories

The design of the operatories is often where my practice is very different from the norm. I'll go into detail now so you can get a feel of what we do at my practice.

Layout

I don't like to have cabinets on the sides of my operatories and I'll tell you why. If you give people a counter, they will clutter it, plain and simple. If you have side cabinets in your operatories, I invite you to start looking through them. How often do you need any of the things you store in there?

Declutter that mess.

My operatories are 8.5" x 10.5". You may think that is small, but I assure you it isn't—if there are no cabinets on the sides. They're clean and clutter free.

I like rear delivery even though, ergonomically, it's not the best choice. I think it's more important that all the instruments and materials are behind the patients, where they don't have to see them and don't get nervous.

Ceiling

Patients are laying back staring at whatever is on your ceiling. You'd better not have dead flies in your lights or a bunch of dust on your air vents. Take this seriously. Remember they are judging your dentistry based on what they see.

I don't like overhead lights. Use a loupe light. Ask anyone who uses one if they would ever go back to the overhead light. With no overhead light, it will free up your ceiling for something even better—a TV!

I can't stress enough how much the patients love the TV's on the ceiling. We used a projector mount to attach the TV to the ceiling. Patients have come to me many times and said that their friend told them about the TV and that is how they heard about us. Pretty soon, this will be the norm, so get those TV's up there ASAP while it is still novel. Also, we run a headphone line from the TV to a pair of headphones. Patients love these! It's a great distraction for patients and especially kids.

Rear Cabinet

Think of this as your workstation. You want everything you need for almost all your procedures back there. Stuff that needs a little more equipment can be placed on a mobile cart. I am talking about endo things, implant things, laser, etc.

Buy extra inventory so that all operatories have the stuff you use the most often. To stock all your ops with the materials will take a larger initial investment in inventory, but never forget what you lose by having to leave the room, not to mention the stress it creates. At my office, each minute I am in the room is worth about $20 in production. Time adds up.

I like to have all my operatories stocked the same with tackle box organizers on the back cabinet. This allows any assistant or hygienist to be comfortable finding things in any room. Every drawer is identical across each operatory as well. This is key to producing efficiently. Evaluate how your rooms are stocked and see what you can do to make it more universal.

Wall

I like to have a second TV on my wall. I purposely have a larger TV on the ceiling than on the wall so that when the patient leans back, they are impressed that it is relatively larger than the wall TV. A lot of the time, the patient doesn't even know the TV is on the ceiling until we lean them back. It is always a good "wow" moment.

My wall TV is hooked up to my computer so that I can use it for treatment presentation. Taking photos and showing them on a screen helps me show my patients what I'm talking about and give them the information they need to trust me and my decisions for their care.

I like the cheap eBay and Amazon cameras. Honestly, they are like $100 as opposed to $3–5k. When they break, you just unplug it and drop it in the trash. The pictures may not be as good as we see on the lecture circuits, but for patient education, they are just fine.

Consult Room

The consult room needs to be somewhere quiet where a staff member can discuss treatment and present financial options. Have it be clutter free and comfortable.

I have my "wall of fame" in my consult room—essentially, it's my diplomas, fellowships, and every certificate I have ever gotten from taking CE. I framed them all and they cover a huge wall. People are impressed by this. My treatment coordinator knows to point out that I take a lot of courses and that I am passionate about dentistry. You can't tell the patients this yourself, or you sound like you are bragging. You need a wall full of plaques and certificates to do that for you.

You may not believe it, but I have won the America's Top

Dentist award every year since I have been open. You know that $150-200 award you can buy? I buy it every year. I'm not sure what criteria the company that makes them uses to decide who wins, but I really don't care. It means something to patients. I have one at my checkout desk, my consult room, my front desk, and my waiting room. Patients occasionally congratulate me on them. It's great!

Sterile Area

If your patients can see this, it needs to look immaculate at all times. Also, talk to your team about improving efficiency in this area by reorganizing or moving some things around.

Mobile Carts

At my office we use mobile carts for a few things. Nitrous, Endo, Ortho, Implants, and our Diode Laser. Each cart has a power strip with a plug coming out the back, so that it can be plugged in and power up everything in the cart with one plug. Endo, for instance, has a lot of different elements that you couldn't possibly stock in every room. Get these things on mobile carts because you never know when endo is about to happen. You need to be able to set up quickly and get that endo rolling if it shows up as an emergency. I had a cabinet maker make my carts, but you can buy these on the internet as well. My ortho cart is from the container store.

11. Your Website

Yes, your website is part of your physical practice. For many prospective patients, it is your 'storefront.' You need quality, professionally done photos of your practice. No, I don't mean your cousin who has a nice camera, or even your friend the realtor. Find a photographer who specializes in the sorts of photos that appear in brochures and on advertising. Photos send a strong message to anyone viewing the site. If they're not balanced, well-framed, in focus and professional, people will decide that your practice is unbalanced, unfocused, and unprofessional. Send the right message about your practice. Hire a professional with experience photographing businesses.

Create Your Environment

The main point to understand here is that your practice should be designed to do two things: provide a great patient experience and allow you to produce efficient dentistry. You control the design of the practice. Although you may be stuck as far as size and walls go, you can decide how to create an environment that sets you up for success. Think about what you'd like to see, do the musical chairs activity with your team, and develop a plan to make your office look like something your patients will talk about. Money spent on an attractive, efficient office is a better use of marketing dollars than money spent on billboards and radio.

Homework

This chapter has a two-part homework assignment, but the parts are linked.

Part 1: Your Staff

Think about your team. Name three people who aren't yet all-stars, but who could be with proper coaching. Write their names down, and a next actionable goal for coaching each. For instance, your receptionist might need phone training. Perhaps your billing person could benefit from CE to help her better understand the procedures you do and proper coding, etc.

Now, think about how you 'Fill their Buckets'. Come up with one bucket-filling action that you plan to take each day this week and write it down. Or, write down the names of your team. This week, when you fill someone's bucket, put a check next to their name. Make sure everyone is getting their buckets filled consistently; without writing it down and checking it off, it's easy to miss someone!

Part 2: Your Brand

What is the current brand identity for your office? Write it down. Now, where does your practice need to improve in expressing this brand identity? Write down three areas where you need to be more on-brand, and what you need to do to make these areas on-brand.

CHAPTER 7
APPROACHING GREATNESS

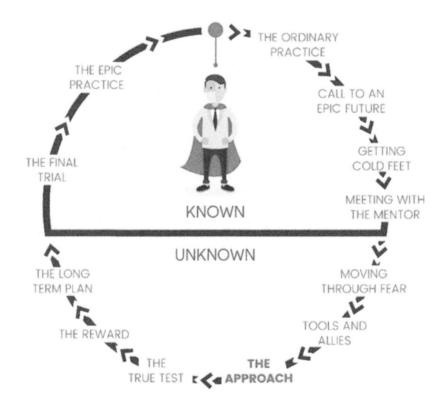

"SUCCESS WITHOUT FULFILLMENT IS THE ULTIMATE FAILURE"

– Tony Robbins

We're getting closer to the real work now, so it's time to stop and reflect for a moment. Why are you on this quest? What final steps do you need to prepare to meet the challenges ahead? What will make your trials worth all the work?

Often, when our peers define success, they do so in monetary terms. Many of our peers see success as a high income, flashy purchases, and a lifestyle that prompts envy in their friends, family, and neighbors.

Our peers are chasing the wrong dream. I was talking to a very popular life and success coach who told me that successful professionals are some of the most miserable people he has ever met, despite all their monetary success. Money cannot bring happiness, but it can buy you the freedom and the time to live a more fulfilled and happy life.

Two years into my practice I had a major breakdown. Stress was killing me. I didn't spend much time with my wife and daughter, and I was consumed with the practice. I hit a point where there were no more goals to check off my list. I had the family, the money, the house, the cars, and finally my own business. My friends told me I was one of the most successful people they knew. All the things I thought I needed to be happy had materialized, and yet I was miserable.

I had reached the end of the rainbow and the gold I found wasn't fulfilling at all.

My closest friends couldn't believe how unhappy I was. "Look at all the things you've got! I wish I had your job or made your kind of money You've got the best wife and a great family!"

My friend Marilee told me of a story in which she once ran a half-marathon in California. It was a really pretty run, great scenery and great weather to go along with it. She couldn't wait for it to begin, but it was a hard race for her. She was tired. She looked down at her shoes the whole time and just kept saying to herself, "Just a little further, just to the top of that hill, just to the bottom of that hill." Once she was done, she was exhausted. She realized later that day that she didn't enjoy the journey of the race. She was so focused on pushing herself to the next goal, that she missed all the beauty happening around her during the run.

Don't miss the beauty in the journey.

Money, by itself, is generally unfulfilling. What's more important is relating to the people sharing our journey. What kind of legacy do you want to leave?

I was miserable because my life lacked balance.

I needed to refocus on what was important to me. I needed a new personal vision. Once I decided that I wanted to spend more time with my family, enjoy my time at work more, and spend less time working, I started to redesign my practice around my personal goals.

I wasn't the hero in my life story until I understood why I was making the journey in the first place.

Retirement is a Lousy Motivator

Something in Tim Ferris's *The Four Hour Work Week* really hit home for me. If you push yourself to work hard for years because you're focused on your retirement, you're making a bad trade. You're trading the years you have now, where you have a chance to have great relationships with your children, to travel, to experience great health and endless possibilities. In return, you get your old age, when it's too late to build relationships with your kids, you're too sick to travel, and you're too worn out to do much of anything, if you even live that long.

Working solely for retirement is a bad deal.

I once heard a story about how a man and his wife saved and saved so they could retire in Colorado and go hiking and climbing every day. They lived a very small life. They were extremely focused on saving for their freedom and retiring at 50. When they were only a few months from retirement, they bought some really nice climbing gear and hiking outfits.

The wife was diagnosed with terminal cancer and died shortly after. The husband retired but no longer wanted to move. He was angry when he looked at the climbing gear that they were going to use in Colorado. He looked at all the years they could have spent hiking and vacationing, enjoying each other. They had hyper-focused on working and saving, and now he had nothing.

Finally, Tim Ferris points out that if you can actually retire early and have enough money to provide a really good life, you're probably a pretty energetic, ambitious, and entrepreneurial person. Do you really think you'd enjoy spending the rest of your life on one long vacation? How do you think a really ambitious person would feel about not having anything to do? You'd be miserable.

A better outcome to strive for is to use dentistry to sustain a life we can enjoy *right now*. We are so blessed to be in a profession that allows us to build businesses that can provide us so many three or four day weekends along with months of vacation time, but only if we choose to take it. That's the kicker right there! You have to take it!

When I considered going down to three days a week, everyone I knew thought I was nuts. "These are your prime production years! You need to put your nose to the grindstone and sock some money away!" I was scared. I feared I'd lose patients and that I wouldn't make enough money to make ends meet. Then I started thinking about the worse vs. best case scenario.

Worst case would be that my income would drop and the practice would begin to decline. I thought about what I would do. It was easy; I would just go back to work another day. Not so bad. What if I lost patients that I needed? I could just do some more marketing and get some new butts in the chairs.

The best case scenario would be that I would still have a good income and have more time to spend with my family and pursuing other interests of mine. I felt like I would likely land somewhere in the middle. I can tell you looking back it was worth it. I won't retire as early as I could if I worked four or five days a week, but I am enjoying life a lot more.

Living in the Middle

Truth is, we will never have the perfect work/life balance. When I say life, I mean family, hobbies, friends, and taking the time off to refuel or as a friend of mine says, "feed the machine." Gary Keller talks about work/life balance in his book, *The One Thing*. He explains that what most people consider as a perfect work/life balance is what he calls "living in the middle". The problem with living in the middle is that nothing extraordinary happens there. It prevents you from making any extraordinary time commitments to either ends of the dichotomy. Sometimes to really take it to the next level at work, the life side of your balance needs to suffer. To take it to the next level in life, sometimes the work side needs to suffer.

Confucius said, "The man who chases two rabbits catches neither." Gary Keller refers to this as "middle mismanagement." The problem is that whenever you focus on anything, something else will be unserved. You will never have true balance. He suggests that when you get out of balance, you never go so far that you cannot come back or that you stay so long so that when you do finally come back, there isn't anything to come back to.

Think of a father who really works hard for a number of years while his children are young and then cuts back so that he can spend more time with them once they're older. They may not even want to be around him after being emotionally abandoned for so long. There is no sense in working so hard that once you finally have that freedom, you have no one to share it with. You can have the freedom now, just not completely, but you will be so much more fulfilled.

Getting your practice in shape will initially mean shifting your balance to the work side, but the result will be a lot more time for the life side of the balance, and a lot more freedom to pursue your personal and professional dreams.

Subtraction over Addition

A major theme I want to stress is that removing stressful things from our lives will bring much more happiness than accumulating more things. I think about how stressful my scheduling used to be, or how my practice used to lack systems and drop the ball on patients all the time. Once I got the systems in place and got my scheduling under control, I was really happy about it.

Think of the things that stress you out, then figure out a way to subtract them from your life. I have a dentist friend that sold a large house because he got overextended in his spending (ever heard of an overextended dentist?). He was initially ashamed when he sold the house, but soon after he told me of how happy he was to have removed the financial stress of owning it. Living stress-free actually made him even happier than the initial thrill of the house purchase had made him.

New things make us happy only for a short while. It's our general day-to-day comfort that matters much more. Life is too short to be stressed. Make it a priority goal to start removing stresses from both your professional and personal life. Write them down, and decipher what will need to happen to reach your goal of making your life as stress free as possible. It may mean you sell your house, or your car, or stop talking to a toxic friend, opt out of a work commitment, leave the HOA board, or end a relationship—who knows? Everyone is different, but the focus needs to be on removing what stresses you out.

Time to Create

Systems will set you free, but you need the time to create them. Getting more time at home initially takes more time at work. You are going to need to go out of balance to set up your business in the manner that affords you time to get away from it.

A major theme of Michael Gerber's, *The E-Myth Revisited*, is that every business needs an Entrepreneur, a Manager, and a Technician. The problem most of us have when we open our practices is that we are only the technician. We are the person producing the product and sales. If we only focus on that aspect, which many dentists are guilty of, we don't properly manage and grow the business.

In Chuck Blakeman's *Making Money is Killing your Business*, he talks about how staying in the production realm and tending to what he calls the *tyranny of the urgent* keeps you from the *priority of the important*. The "important" is creating the systems that set you free from the business and allow it to make money without you there.

The problem is that we stay in the technician role, too busy working on the urgent things to ever take the time to set up the systems that make our lives easier in the long run.

Aspire to Delegation

To have time to build the business, you need to learn to delegate effectively.

That means you need to realize where you get the most bang for your buck at the practice. For the dentist, this will be cutting teeth, tissues, bone, or taking things out of them. That means not making temporaries, not designing your own CEREC's, not taking photos or gathering records, writing lab slips, packaging cases, etc.

Those tasks need to be done by your trained team. Delegating gives you more time to be working on teeth, making you more efficient at work.

What about writing notes, doing payroll, paying vendors, scanning receipts, and bookkeeping? You shouldn't be doing those either. You need to train team members on those as well. If you can delegate all of your non-cutting practices to someone else, you will have the time to work at creating the business systems that will give you freedom.

Training someone takes a lot of time up front, but that commitment pays off long term. The more time you have free, the more time you have to train other staff members and delegate. It's a time snowball. Once a team member is trained on something, they can then train someone else and the snowball grows laterally into something like a giant snow hot dog.

Delegating is hard, especially when we're good at something. But remember, you don't need to go to dental school to learn how to do most of the things that happen at the dental practice. Try delegating and make adjustments as you go.

"Ready, Fire, Aim!"

The Time is Now

One of the hardest things about pursuing a goal is getting started. Make the commitment right now that you are going to begin moving toward de-stressing your life and decreasing your nonproductive workload at the office. Do not take this step lightly.

Think about two prisoners with life sentences that constantly talk and dream about escaping prison and getting their freedom back. They talk and talk, planning relentlessly for years, but they are both just talkers until the moment one of them finally decides to start digging a hole. Break out of your practice prison; start digging your hole.

Homework

What are three tasks in the practice that you currently delegate? Write them down, who they're delegated to, and what sort of results you're getting.Now, write down the top three tasks you wish you could delegate. What are they? Who could you delegate them to? If it's a team member, write down what step you need to take next to be able to delegate.

If you need to contract them out, write down the name of the staff member who will be in charge of researching contractors and contacting them about demos and quotes.

CHAPTER 8
THE TRUE TEST — SYSTEMS ARE EVERYTHING

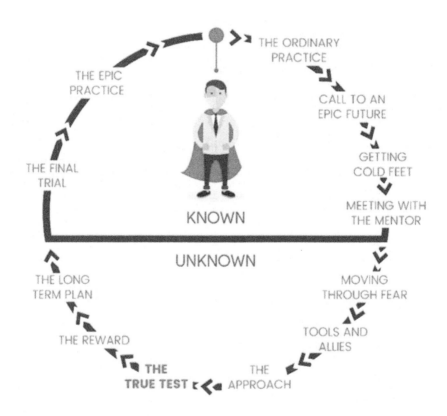

Create the Systems that Set You Free

Webster defines a system as "a set of principles or procedures according to which something is done; an organized scheme or method". For our purposes, we will define a system as the way we Get Things Done. Mentally, I call it GSD, where I substitute another, more accurate, word for 'things.'

Systems are not created overnight. They are the product of trial and error, and unfortunately a lot of times, unhappy patients. If you have a culture of coachability where everyone is free to fail and be honest about it, you can discuss those failures and create systems that prevent them from happening again. As you become busier everyone will be juggling a lot of balls at the practice. When those balls start to fall, you know that's a place to create a system.

There are seven major system categories that control everything in the office. Before you can begin to create and refine those systems, you need a method for creating new systems. That begins with communication between you and the team.

Team Meetings Help You Plan Your Attack

In order to create and implement systems, you need to discuss them. Team meetings are the easiest way to have a whole-practice discussion about new systems and get them implemented.

At my first associateship, there was a single meeting in the entire three-year period that I worked there. It turned into a staff meltdown. People were angry, and with good reason. The back blamed the front, the front blamed the back, the doctors blamed the management and the supply ordering, etc. It was awful. They never had another meeting.

Meltdowns like that happen when team concerns don't have a constructive outlet, when there's no way for staff to approach practice managers with suggestions, and when people bottle up their frustrations for a long time. I suggest weekly to bi-weekly meetings while you are implementing a lot of things, and then hold them monthly once things are running smoothly.

My practice has monthly meetings for an hour and a half and then quarterly meetings in which we spend four hours breaking out into different departments (hygiene, front office, assistants) and really discussing what we can improve upon and how we are going to implement it. After the meeting, we do something fun like all go bowling, paintballing, whirly ball, etc. Sometimes we hold our monthly meetings at the practice, and sometimes we all go out to a restaurant. It's good to vary things a bit so that they don't become boring and routine.

I like to keep a running note in my phone for the team meeting. That way I can enter ideas easily and quickly as they arise during the month. Simply saying to yourself, "I need to remember to bring that up at the next meeting," is not enough. You can even have a sheet somewhere in your practice where anyone can write down meeting topics as they think of them.

A lot of doctors will gripe about shutting down production and paying their team for meetings, but I assure you it is money well spent. Your greatest return on investment will come from having a great team working together in harmony.

Morning huddles give everyone a chance to look at the day together and see if anything special will need to be done. They're a way to plan in advance how everyone will stay on-brand in difficult interactions and a reminder about what systems are in place. You can look at spots where you will need a little help, talk about patients with balances, or talk about what needs to happen with a case. Don't just ramble off a bunch of BS numbers no one cares about. Talk about things that are useful to plan and implement your day.

Don't forget that the whole purpose of systems is so that things run well.

Any new system you create can be tested, refined, and evaluated. I know there are many systems in my practice that I don't even know about, mainly on the front office side of things.

If a system isn't working, I find out because something fails. Then my team and I come up with a new system so that it doesn't happen again. That's how you create great systems!

Checklists are Your Weapon in the Fight Against Error

Checklists are a must for great systems. We have checklists for check in, check out, morning, middle day, and nighttime duties; attending to recall and unscheduled treatment lists; weekly and monthly maintenance; etc. Most of these checklists are initialed by someone and placed on my desk. The great thing about checklists is they create accountability.

For example, we used to say the assistants would tidy up the lab and break room before going home, but it didn't always get done. Once we added a checklist that was placed on my desk before leaving, I could see if the tasks had been completed. If they weren't, but someone had initialed them, I knew who I had to talk to.

Nobody leaves at night until the whole checklist is done.

Something to know about checklists is that you have to check up and audit them. Only the things you audit will get done. If your staff realizes you never really notice when things don't get completed, their motivation to get those things completed goes down significantly.

The Most Important Illustration in this Book

I created the illustration below to help you understand schematically how patients move through the practice and generate income. This is a schematic that lets you see the places where you and your team may need more training, more clearly defined protocols, or more detailed systems in place to keep your practice on-brand and running from day-to-day.

When you are clear about how you do things, you don't have to intervene a lot. The practice runs smoothly and you can spend your time on high-production procedures or high-level planning instead of dealing with constant crises and drama.

DENTAL OFFICE SALES PROCESS

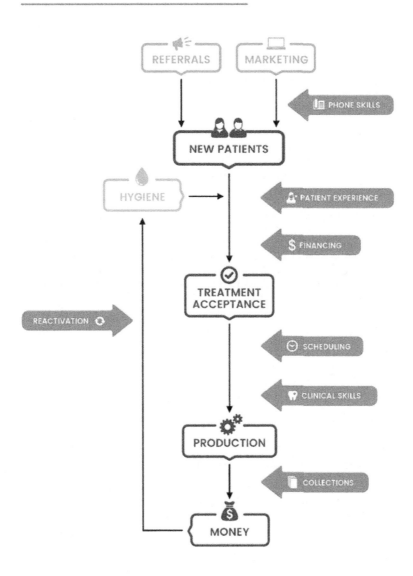

As I see it, there are seven general areas in which you need great systems. These are the arrows in the illustration.

1. Phone Skills
2. Patient Experience
3. Financing
4. Scheduling
5. Clinical Skills
6. Collections
7. Reactivation and Recall

Focus on these areas to transform your practice. These are the areas where you should be collecting statistics and setting clear goals. If your practice is falling short of your expectations, these are the places that you're failing. Training needs to center on these categories.

Look at the diagram and think about how a patient moves through each of these categories in your practice. Move through each category, tracking the current process and finding places where you're failing your team, your patients, or your business.

Where are the snags in your current process? You have a system already, even if you haven't codified it. However, your current system probably has snags and gaps. Focus in on those gaps, and, as a team, brainstorm improvements.

Once you break things down and create clear-cut systems for each area, you start to see improvement across the board. So, you can make improvements in scheduling and see improvement in collections. You can make improvements in your clinical skills by getting more training or becoming more efficient; you can improve your collections procedures by having clear policies in place. All the meat and potatoes comes down to this diagram and asking, "What are we going to do in these seven areas?"

To create a cohesive, on-brand experience for your patients and your staff, you need systems to move the patient through the practice, provide great care at each touchpoint, and ensure that you have happy patients who want to refer others to your practice. Happy, appreciative patients are what make the practice a great place to work for your team, and a happy team is what makes for happy, appreciative patients.

Clear systems create a brand-experience feedback loop that leads to a great practice.

The Practice Growth Cycle

Have you ever known someone who is in high-intensity training for an athletic event like a triathlon or weightlifting competition? If you talk to these top athletes, they use the word 'plateau' a lot. A typical training regimen involves time where abilities increase rapidly, and then times where the increase stops. The athlete isn't losing ground, but he's stopped gaining new ground. He needs to break though some barrier to take his performance to the next level.

The same thing happens when you're trying to expand your dental practice. You have ideas, discuss them, implement them, and then reevaluate and develop new ideas from your experiences. (Remember Ready, Fire, Aim? That applies here too.) That cycle provides the momentum that will carry your practice to the next level. But once you reach that level, you're at a plateau. You need even more energy, some bigger change, to start growing again.

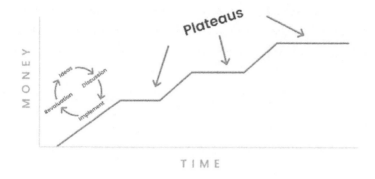

As you begin to discuss and implement new systems with your team, you will begin to see growth to a point at which you cannot grow anymore. That will be your plateau. In my experience, these happened at my practice at $85k a month, $110k a month, $150k a month, and where we are now, at about $230K a month.

At each of these plateau points, you hit capacity. This means your schedules are full, you are busy, and you cannot make any more money under the current conditions. This is a good place to be. Plateaus are pivot points. You can make big decisions about whether you want to keep growing, or whether you'd rather refine what you have.

Think of your practice as a cup full of water. The cup has a finite capacity. Once that cup is full, you either have to make the cup larger (increase capacity) or substitute wine for the water (increase value of existing capacity).

You can increase capacity by adding new operatories, chairs, associates, days, etc. Substituting wine for the water would be things like pulling off of fee schedules, raising your fees, scheduling more productively, or having more strict policies, such as prepayment of appointments. Either way, you have to work within the existing constraints of your cup.

If our number one goal is growing our practices, we can't

ignore the practice growth cycle. We want to reach the plateaus. We want to get to where we can't produce any more dollars with our current systems.

Good systems drive growth so that you can reach a new plateau. To move beyond that, you either need to create new systems or apply old systems with increased capacity. So, every time we hit a plateau, we should be excited, because that means we have gotten the most out of our current systems and we are ready for the next step in our growth. The next step will be unique to you and your personal and professional goals. But, before you are ready for that next step, you need to first reach that plateau.

Every time my practice hits a plateau, I say to myself, "I don't know how we can possibly do any more in revenue." We discuss the current state of the practice as a team, refine our systems, and then continue to take the practice to another level.

The systems, and refining them, drive the growth. It's Ready, Fire, Aim, all over again. It means making changes. Whatever you decide, your heroic leadership is what's going to get your staff and your practice through the change and onto a higher level.

Homework

All right, it's time to put pen to paper on the seven areas for systems. But you're not going to be able to do this by sitting in a chair, and it's not going to be fast.

- Get out your calendar and plan to look at one system category a day for the next seven business days.

- Look at how they work, and don't work, at busy times and slow times.

- Write down the current system, and circle where things are failing.

- Have a few trusted team members do the same. Often different people will spot different fail points and chokepoints.

- On the eighth day, sit down and discuss where your systems are failing.

- Reconvene in a week to come up with solutions.

- Create new systems AND TRAIN YOUR STAFF ON THEM. This is very important. It's easy to fall back into old patterns, and simply posting a system on the wall won't make it a reality. Train first, then post the system and remind people about them.

- Expect changes. Many things look great on paper but hit roadblocks in the real world. Frank Lloyd Wright's houses are gorgeous, but notoriously difficult to maintain or live in. Systems are like this too. Be humble, and be ready to change to find the perfect system for each of the seven areas in your practice.

CHAPTER 9
THE TRUE TEST—MARKETING TO WIN

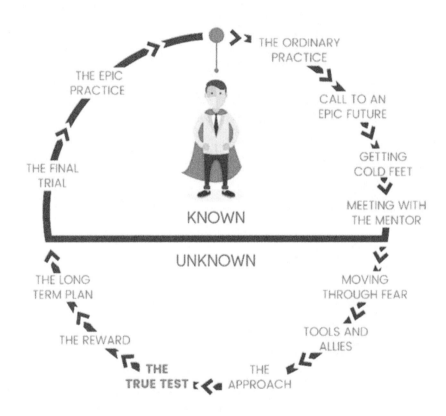

In order to increase new patients and get us closer to our capacity point, we need to market. Marketing needs to be a budget item in a growing practice. Anywhere from 2–8% of your collections should be designated for marketing, depending on where you are at in your growth.

Due to regular and expected attrition for a practice, the rule is that somewhere around 20-25 new patients per full-time doctor per month will keep active patients stable, while anything less is indicative of a practice in decline. Anything more is a practice in a growth phase.

We want to go big into growth until we reach our capacity point, or production plateau. At that point, we will need to either increase capacity or increase value.

You get a lot of advertising from companies promising dentists insane numbers of new patients a month by way of external marketing. What I want to emphasize is that external marketing is important to get new patients in the door, but it can only bring you so many. What really gets you to the point of treating 100 new patients a month (which is a crazy amount) is having the great patient experience and systems that generate new patients from your existing ones.

Think of it this way. If your external marketing can bring in around 25 patients per month, you should be able to generate an additional three people per new patient from those patients.

How you ask?

If we say that each family on average has 2.5–3 people in it, we want to make sure we schedule the rest of the family when the first member comes to our office as a new patient. We also hope that they will refer at least one other person to our practice. This can be someone they work with or an extended family member. The goal is to generate, on average, three additional people from your one new patient. If you do this with 25 new patients one month, you will see an additional 75 new patients from that 25.

If your patient experience is top notch, it's not hard to get these referrals. They just happen organically. All you have do, other than wow your new patients on their first visit, is make sure that you schedule their immediate family members, and the rest is history.

If you fail to impress the patient on the first visit, you will have a hard time getting large growth numbers. If your patients don't find your office remarkable enough to talk about or send additional family members to, you're not going to generate large new patient numbers. Those new patients may not even stay in your practice themselves.

The key is to maximize those on-brand interactions and to make sure that each and every touchpoint provides a great experience. Remember, dental patients come in with pretty low expectations, so it only takes a bit of thought and effort on your part to turn them into brand ambassadors for your office.

There was a two-year point in which we stopped external marketing efforts completely. We still continued to see around 80 new patients every month. We were at a capacity point and could barely fit anyone in. New patients would wait sometimes four months to get in to us for a COE.

That's the power of patient experience.

So, you're ready to market, and you've got the systems in place to support the effects of your marketing. The three most important avenues of marketing for dentists are:

- Online marketing and reputation management
- Mailers
- Location and signage

There are, of course, other avenues, and everyone practices in different areas, so results may vary. For my practice, these have brought the most ROI.

Avenue 1: Online Marketing and Reputation Management

The greatest new patient source I have, other than word of mouth, comes from dominating Google searches. Before the internet, people asked family for recommendations when they needed a new dentist. Nowadays, they may start by asking their cousin, but they'll double check the recommendation by checking your office out on Facebook or Googling you.

Plan on spending anywhere from four to seven thousand dollars for a website that has the sort of content, formatting, and metadata that Google likes. It's money well spent. If you are number one on Google searches for your area, you can easily expect 20-30 new patients a month, depending on the size of your town, the number of dentists, etc. You won't get a larger ROI in any other external marketing, I promise.

Be wary of "dental" website companies. A lot of these have the same content across multiple sites but just change the practice name and colors. Google loves original content. Having duplicate content can hurt your rankings.

Let Them Get to Know You

The most read page on your website will be your "Meet the Doctor" page. You need to make this palatable. A short paragraph about where you went to school is not enough. You need to write about your interests and who you are as a person. You also need to have a picture. The patients want to see the doctor. Get a nice picture taken by a professional and get it updated every so many years. Have a picture of your family on your page. Show yourself doing things in your community or abroad. Put up pictures of yourself engaged in your hobbies. If you have a dull and boring, "Meet the Doctor" page, potential patients will go to the next dental website in your area in an attempt to find someone who's not just a 'generic dentist'—someone they can connect with. If that doctor has an attractive "Meet the Doctor" page, guess whose practice they're going to. Have a "Meet the Team" page where the prospective patient can learn more about the team members. Again, get professional pictures taken with everyone in the same scrub colors.

Films Have Power

Another aspect of your website that helps convert patients is video. You can get testimonials from existing patients and post them to YouTube. You can then link to them from your website.

You can also hire a production firm to come out and make a short one minute video showcasing your practice. This works really well when you have a great practice to showcase, so start with that. These can run anywhere from $1000-3000 to create. I know that's a lot to spend, but if we consider that a new patient may be worth around $1000 (many consultants say more), a nicely produced video more than pays for itself if they can convert only one to three patients in the lifetime that you use it. And, let's be honest, it is going to convert a lot more patients than that.

Finally, make sure your phone number is large and visible on every page of your site. It should also be clickable, so patients can click to dial from their mobile phones. After all, that is the ultimate goal of the website: to create a phone call to your practice.

The website creates the first impression of what your office is like for the patient. It's the first touchpoint where you can express your brand identity. Take it seriously and execute it well. Hire the right people and spend the money to get your website looking top notch. It's worth every penny.

Reviews Lead to Page Views

Ask your patients to review your practice on Google. It only takes a few moments, and since Google is the most dominant search engine, Google reviews are the most important reviews. Google "your town" and dentist. You want to be on the top three, as you will display at the top of the organic results as well as the "local" or "map" page. Reviews appear next to the name of the top three practices.

If you live in an area where Yelp reviews also carry a lot of weight, focus your efforts there as well.

If you have more stars and more reviews than your competitors, users will be drawn to your site. If you don't have reviews or all you have is negative ones, don't worry about your website, because no one is going to it.

That is why it is a key element of a great practice to solicit these reviews. You can give the team bonuses if you want to get everyone involved.

There are many software packages that allow you to send a review request to your patients after they visit you. But what will really tip the scales is if you ask for them personally, as the dentist.

You don't have to ask everyone, but if any patient gives you a compliment, you can say something like, "Thank you so much! You know what, it would really help us grow if you would go on Google and write us an online review. Could you do that for me?" They will always say yes. Then you send them the email or text request. They are much more likely to follow through if the doctor personally asks for it.

Learn to Handle Negative Reviews

You are bound to get some negative reviews. That's ok; you just need to have many more positive ones than negative ones. If you get a negative review, don't get defensive in your online response—it only makes you look worse.

Instead, practice giving responses like this: "We are so sorry that you had a negative experience with us. 100% patient satisfaction is a strong element of our practice. I'd love to talk to you personally about how we can make this right. If you are interested, great! If not, I hope you find a new dentist that can continue to care for your teeth, because that is what is most important. We would be happy to forward along your records should you request it. I hope to speak to you soon!"

You may be biting a hole through your tongue as you type a response like that, but if you start defending yourself online in response to a negative review, it makes you look like the jerk the reviewer just described. Always take the high road.

SEO, Social Media, and Pay-per-Click

SEO, or search engine optimization, is becoming more and more powerful and the rules are changing every day. Don't handle this on your own unless you have a designated in-house person with dedicated time to work on it. Otherwise, pay the experts.

You need to be active on social media and advertising. You also need to think about pay-per-click advertisements. There are a lot of companies that will provide all-encompassing online marketing for you. Get some referrals from people you know who are doing it well.

I always ask the companies to give updates on what they're doing for me. There are a lot of scam SEO and online marketing people out there. You want to see that they are writing original content, checking what ads are working and what are not, and making regular updates to your website. If they can't show you what they've done, find someone else.

Avenue 2: Mailers

For mailers to be effective, you have to use them correctly. This is where many dentists fail.

A successful mail piece needs three elements:

- It is large
- It highlights one or two marketable attributes or benefits to the patient
- It hits the household at least three times

Large Postcards

When you price out postcard printing and postage, you will see that very large postcards cost more money. It's often a couple thousand more for the same number of mail pieces. If you consider that an average new patient is worth a thousand dollars, the extra money is worth it. You want your mailer to stand out from all the other junk mail that comes along. Spend the money, and don't get seduced by the cheap mailers that come along with the local discount magazine. One, you don't want patients who shop primarily on price, and two, your piece won't get seen.

Highlight Only One or Two Marketable Attributes

The primary purpose of a mailer is to generate a new patient phone call. Too much information will only confuse prospective patients. Pick one or two things to highlight, such as late hours, a high tech practice, patient comfort, or same-day crowns. Don't list every procedure you provide; get more focused. Sit down with your team and think about what is marketable about your practice. If you can't think of anything, that may be a big part of your problem.

Use actual pictures. My most effective mail piece that I send out has three pictures on the front, all taken by a professional. One is of my waiting room. The second picture is of our "kids room." It has a caption underneath it that reads, "The kids can play in our kid-only room!" The third picture is of the TV's on the ceiling. This picture has a caption that reads, "Watch TV while we clean your teeth!" That's it. Three enticing pictures on a big post card.

Compare that to what prospective patients usually receive: a small post card, with generic stock photography that says, "Accepting new patients!"

This type of mailer markets nothing.

Their mailer essentially only says that one, we are a dental office, and two, we are accepting new patients. These kind of mailers aren't marketing your practice, they're marketing 'generic dentist.'

Hit Each Household at Least Three Times

Direct mail marketing has to be repeated to be effective. Hit each address at least three times. Also, if your mailers have consistent color schemes and look alike, they will always build upon each other. These should be the same colors on your logo, website, and any other print you have.

Mailers need to reinforce your brand identity.

Make sure that you split your mailing to drop one quarter each week. This way if you generate a lot of calls you don't have one week where the phones are going crazy. Spread the mailer out over a month. All direct mail companies can do this if you ask.

Mailers need to have a call to action, but avoid loss leaders. Loss leaders are when you advertise a service very cheap to get a patient in the door, such as $29 cleanings. You will rarely get great patients with this kind of tactic. It also cheapens your office. We want to create a brand that people are willing to pay for. Don't be seduced by competing on price; it's like crack to the consumer and once they are hooked, and you stop giving them cheap crack, they will leave your office in search of cheaper crack without blinking an eye.

Avenue 3: Location and Signage

You've heard it before, "location, location, location!" We need to place our offices in areas that are visible to traffic passing by. If someone passes your office on their way to work, they likely pass it on the way back, and on the way to the grocery store, and on the way to the mall, etc. That's a lot of exposures. But if they can't see your practice because you are tucked inside a professional building, they won't know you exist. You may save a little on rent, but you'll lose out on new patients. How many new patients could you grab if you were visible? Could you grab one or two more? Could you then see their family members and friends and get another six to eight patients out of it? Yes. Pay the money for the visible space. Being visible from the street is huge. It will work synergistically with all of your other marketing efforts to bring in new patients. When we first opened, we were seeing around 20 or so new patients a month that put "drive by" as their referral source. That's powerful.

Give Me a Sign!

Get the biggest sign that your landlord and city will allow, and then spend the money for it. A large sign will give you way more exposure and ROI than any other form of marketing. Make sure it lights up and stands out. Make sure it is readable from the street.

What's in a Name?

What did you name your practice? Did you just put your name there? Don't do that. If someone driving by wants to Google you, your practice name will be hard to remember and hard to spell. Think of a creative name for your practice. We named ours after the adjacent neighborhood and middle school down the street.

The most laughable dental signage I see is when it just says in red block letters, "DENTIST". All this says is that you are ordinary, just like every other dentist. Create a brand with a great name. When you put it on your sign, make sure that "Dental" or "Family Dental" is the larger portion. Don't let the first part of your practice name drown out the dental part. The dental part is the part that needs to be the most visible, so that people know that you're a dental office. For example, picture a sign that says "NELSON RIDGE" in very large visible letters and then in really small letters underneath says, "FAMILY DENTAL." Someone driving by may pass that sign their entire life and never know what "NELSON RIDGE" actually sold because the second part was so small they couldn't read it from the street.

If your office has a bad sign, drop a few thousand on a better one. It will be worth it.

Homework

It's time to do an online marketing tune-up. Sit down with your computer. Now, visit the website and social media accounts for your practice. What do you see? Write down the first thing that jumps out at you on each page, what you like, what you don't, what seems counterintuitive or confusing. Have someone you know do the same. Pretend that you're different kinds of patients: a parent, someone with an emergency, someone who needs major reconstructive work. Does the page speak to you and make it easy to find information?

Write down any ideas you have for improving the page.

Now, do a Google search for *Yourtown* Dentist. Which sites come up? Visit the top three sites that aren't yours, and go through the same process. Visit their social media pages too. Why might someone searching online choose their practice over yours?

CHAPTER 10
THE TRUE TEST—NOW THE PHONE IS RINGING

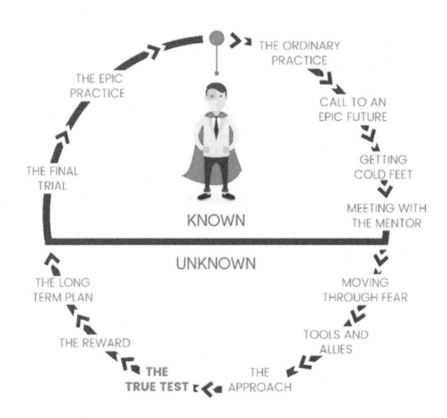

THE ORDINARY
PRACTICE

THE EPIC
PRACTICE

CALL TO AN
EPIC FUTURE

THE FINAL
TRIAL

GETTING
COLD FEET

KNOWN

MEETING WITH
THE MENTOR

UNKNOWN

THE LONG
TERM PLAN

MOVING
THROUGH FEAR

THE REWARD

TOOLS AND
ALLIES

THE
TRUE TEST

THE
APPROACH

Some people say that their marketing isn't working because they aren't getting any new patients. Marketing's job is to generate the phone call. Converting the call to a new patient is the job of the person answering the phone. If your marketing is generating phone calls but new patient appointments aren't being put on the books, the problem is the phone skills, not the marketing.

Even worse than bad phone skills is not answering the phone at all. If a new patient calls your office and no one picks up, they won't leave a message. They'll hang up and call the next office on Google. The phone must be answered at all costs. Place phones in strategic areas in the practice so that this can be accomplished by the clinical people in the back when all the front office people are already on the phone.

There are entire seminars devoted to phone training. Usually they come from one of two different schools of thought on how a new patient phone call should be handled. One school teaches that we should get the patient in at all costs as quickly as possible and get off the phone. The other is to use that first new patient phone call to build rapport and start creating value and expectations for the office. I believe we should be somewhere in between. We want to get the patient in and we don't want to be on the phone chatting for long periods of time; but we also don't want the whole phone call to be a scripted lifeless process that just makes an appointment.

You Can't Count on the NSA to Track Your Calls

You need phone monitoring for two reasons: the first is to see when and if any phone calls are being missed. Have the culture at your practice that you will not miss any phone calls. Don't allow front desk people to take their breaks at the same time. Don't schedule lunch for when you usually have the largest volume of calls. This is usually around 11:30-1:00 at my office.

Three Rings Max

Have a phone at every desk, and a cordless phone in the clinical area so that if no one in front can answer the phone, you or the clinical staff can grab the cordless. If answering every phone call is important to you, it will become important to the team as well. Have the policy that the phone needs to be answered within two rings. If it rings a third time, anyone who hears it better come running down that hall and pick it up. Sometimes I have to grab the cordless and run it down the hall to someone. You might wonder why I don't answer it myself. I did it once; it was so strange that I'll never do it again. Remember, you often only get one chance to answer that new patient call, so don't blow it by letting it go to a machine. Often, an office can increase their new patients solely by just answering the phone more consistently.

Even if the doctor is not at the office, staff should always be there to field phone calls. Someone needs to be at your office from Monday through Friday from 9 to 5 at the bare minimum. Even better would be having someone take a forwarded cell phone home or stay later and come in on Saturdays to take phone calls. It doesn't take a whole lot of after-hour new patient calls for it to be worth it. If a new patient is worth $1000, a $15 per hour employee would have to convert just one new patient every 66 hours they work to break even. Check your phone records to see if you are missing calls. I promise it will be an eye-opening experience.

Listen and Learn

The second reason to have phone monitoring software is to listen to and evaluate your team's phone skills. Listening to phone calls is one of my least favorite things to do, but it is critical that you do it. I have an evaluation sheet that I complete and then talk to the team member about their recent phone calls and how close they were to how I want them to be.

If your team knows you might be listening, they will do a better job on the phone. Also, having them listen to themselves is always an eye-opening experience for them. I remember when I wore a wrist watch recorder for a little while and recorded my speaking during my exams. I spoke fast and I cut people off. I had no idea I was doing these things, because sometimes in the moment it there are just too many things going on to notice. When you listen to recordings of yourself, it really helps you to see how you can improve.

Now that you're recording your call, let's look at what it should sound like.

Anatomy of a Call: The Greeting

When someone answers the phone, they should be smiling. The patient will be able to hear that on the other end. That's right, I said they will hear the smile. It's hard to sound unhappy on the phone when you are smiling. Does your front office staff ever get stressed during the day? I bet they do. The front office is required to multitask constantly! Make sure they know to take a breath and smile before picking up that phone. You never get another chance to make that first impression. The greeting will set the tone for the rest of the call.

Greeting your caller enthusiastically and friendly is step one. If your angry and depressed mother-in-law is working your front desk, you may have a problem.

Once I was trying to find somewhere to have LASIK done. I started reading reviews on Google and found one office that had mostly negative reviews. I would say out of eight reviews for this particular office, six were one star, and four of those six directly referenced the woman at the front desk named Diane. If four people wrote directly about Diane, think about how many other patients might have thought she was rude but didn't take the time to post a negative review about it. Remember it only takes one bad apple to be the case killer at the practice. I didn't even call this office, but I pray that the owner has the common sense to fire Diane, get her off the phone, or get her some training.

Answer your phone by saying your practice name and the name of the person answering the phone. We like to say, "Thank you for calling Nelson Ridge Family Dental, my name is _____, and I can help you!" That's right, "*I can help you*".

I once called Six Month Smiles and that was how they answered the phone. Sometime later I had an issue with an order where we ordered the wrong things and had opened them. I thought to myself, "Well, we can't return them now." But then I thought of how they answered the phone, "I can help you." I thought, "If a company says that when they answer the phone, they must really care about taking care of their customers. I bet they will take care of this for me." Wouldn't you know it, they did.

That day we changed the way we answered our phones.

I wanted to convey that level of customer service to my patients the first time they called my office. It is *different*, and in the customer service world, *different* is a great place to be.

Anatomy of a Call: Thank the Patient

Be grateful that they called your office. Thank them immediately! We once switched cleaning services at my home. The new woman always thanked us for the opportunity to clean our house every time she came. She was truly grateful that we chose her. It really made an impact on the way my wife and I feel about her.

We should express that same level of gratefulness to our patients when they call us. It does not take a lot of effort to say,

"Thank you so much for calling our practice!" or "We really appreciate you calling us!" It's also a great segue into the next part of the new patient call: getting the patient's name.

Anatomy of a Call: Get the Patient's Name

Never forget that the greatest word anyone will hear is their own name. You want to use this to your advantage to make the patient feel good and make the call more personal. Get the patient's name early, and use it a few times during your conversation.

Anatomy of a Call: Take Control

The longer you let the patient ask all the questions, the more likely you are to say something stupid. Jay Geher of Scheduling Institute refers to this as "verbal vomit." It happens anytime a team member is asked a difficult question and answers it poorly.

To take control of the call, you simply need to ask the caller a question. If the caller asked you a question, answer it briefly and then before the patient has a chance to ask you another question, ask them something.

The easiest thing to ask is how they found out about the office. What's important is that you start asking the questions, and then listen. A typical new patient call should take anywhere from three to five minutes. It should be short, but remember, it is the first opportunity to start adding value to your dental practice. It should be a positive and memorable experience for the patient. If you take control of the call early with tact and consideration, you can keep the call short while maintaining great customer service to the patient.

If you don't take control of the call, you may find yourself listening to a patient on the phone ramble about something very unimportant. You are now at their mercy. Take control immediately and you can steer the direction of the call while remaining friendly and helpful.

Anatomy of a Call: The Empathy/Value/Hope Statement

We want to give the vibe that our practice cares about our patients. A very easy way to do this is through what I call an **empathy/value/hope** statement. Any time a patient expresses that they are in pain, had a bad experience at another office, or even is having a bad day, we need to reply with an empathy/value/hope statement that says we understand (empathy), they chose the right dental office (value), and that we are going to help them (hope).

The **empathy** part is just acknowledging what is bothering the patient. These are statements like, "I know how you feel," "That sounds awful," or "I would feel the same if that happened to me." There are many ways to do this, but the main point is that you need to express empathy for whatever the patient is feeling.

The **value** statement always follows the empathy statement. This is something that showcases your practice and makes the patient glad they called. In my office, it usually takes the form of making the patient feel better about choosing your office. Statements like, "Doctor is great with toothaches," or "You chose the right place!"

The last part is the **hope** statement. This gives the patient hope that you are moving them to a solution to their problem. These are statements like: "Let's get you in so you can feel better!" or "We need to see you right away so you can get some relief!" The hope statement is the close. You are asking the patient to book an appointment. Ask and you shall receive, so get your staff comfortable asking for the close.

Remember, the new patient or emergency call should be

memorable. The **empathy/value/hope** statement is a critical part of the process.

Here are some scripted examples:

Patient: I have a tooth that is killing me that I need to have looked at.
Staff: Oh my, that sounds awful! Tooth pain is the worst! (Empathy). It's a good thing you called us (Value). Let's get you in to see the doctor today so that we can get you feeling better! (Hope)

Patient: I am calling to switch to your office because I had a really big problem at my previous dentist with them billing me for things they didn't tell me I was going to have to pay.
Staff: I totally know how you feel, I hate when places do that! (Empathy) At our office, we're a little different. We always explain in detail all the charges our patients can expect so there are never surprises (Value). Let's get you an appointment here soon so you can see what I mean (Hope).

Patient: My last dentist drilled too deep and the tooth has been sensitive ever since. He adjusted the bite a few times but it isn't getting any better. I don't think he knows what he is doing.
Staff: Oh my, I get what you mean. Sensitive teeth can sure be a nuisance! (Empathy) The doctor here is great! (Value) Let's get you in to see our doctor so he can take a look and get that tooth feeling better. (Hope)

Patients who are upset with a previous dental office are the easiest to convert because they are seeking an office that will understand them and provide them a solution for where the previous office failed. Let's face it; the majority of our new patients left a previous dental office because of something they did not like. The **empathy/value/hope** statement conveys positive things about your practice and moves the patient to scheduling an appointment.

Anatomy of a Call: Scheduling the Appointment

Give the patient two or three choices when scheduling appointments. Don't ever ask the patient what time they would like to come in. This can lead to a long back and forth process trying to find the absolutely most convenient time for the patient. Instead, ask them, "Would you like a morning, afternoon, or evening appointment?" It's important to note that this is not a yes or no question, it is an either/or. After they tell you what part of the day they would like to come in, give them two options; if they can't do either, they will ask for a different day or just say no. Then give them two other options. The main idea is not to get into the cycle of the patient asking if they can come here and here and you saying no over and over again. Providing alternatives keeps you in control of the call.

Anatomy of a Call: Setting Expectations

After scheduling a time, the staff member on the phone should set the expectations for the patient about their upcoming visit. This means explaining to the patient what will happen at the visit and what will not.

One of my biggest pet peeves is when a new patient comes in and needs a molar root canal, and they are upset that I don't have an hour or so available in my schedule right then and there to do the procedure. They will huff and puff saying, "Uggghhhhh, I told the girl on the phone that I wanted the tooth fixed tonight, I can't believe she didn't schedule it that way!" The time I would have needed to complete that root canal was booked solid well over two or three weeks ago, but patients don't understand that.

The team member who took the call should have explained that we are going to only look at the tooth to see what it needs. If it is a quick fix we may be able to take care of it today, but if it needs more time we will likely set up an appointment to complete the treatment at a later date and will prescribe medicine to help in the meantime. The team member should always also express that we have a full schedule and that we are squeezing them in, so that they understand why we can't always treat them on the same day.

The same goes for new patients coming in for routine hygiene and exam. They should know whether or not they are going to get their teeth cleaned, that we will be taking the necessary x-rays, that the doctor will do an exam, and that we will present all finances and set up times to complete any additional treatment.

Patients get upset when we fail to meet their expectations.

If we do not set the patient's expectations, they will set their own and we may end up not meeting them. For a consistent positive experience, take the time to set the expectations on the phone call.

Anatomy of a Phone Call: Promote the Office

After setting expectations, it's important to talk up the doctor and the office. Everyone on your team should know what courses you take, what fellowships you have, where you went to school, and that you are a great doctor. You know that you are great and you want the patient to think that as well. But if you come into the operatory bragging about all your achievements, it will not come across favorably to the patient. Let your staff do that bragging for you.

An essential part of the phone call is telling the patient that they are going to love the practice and that the doctor is wonderful. Build it up! Don't be afraid to talk about all the extra courses the doctor takes or mission trips that he or she has attended. You need to talk highly about the practice and the doctor because it sets the tone for the visit before the patient even comes in. We want to prime that "patient experience pump" so to speak. Never miss an opportunity to build value.

Anatomy of a Call: Dealing with Price Shoppers

Some of the most difficult questions we get asked on the phone are about money. "How much does a crown cost?" I truly believe that most people don't buy dentistry based on price, yet the question needs to be answered. My staff gives a range.

I don't ever want to give an actual price for two reasons: one, the patient will likely hold that in their mind as an agreement, and two, it gives the caller what they were looking for so that they can hang up and call another office. Always give a range, never a single price. Try to express that there is no way to give an actual price over the phone as there are many variables. For instance, if a caller asks how much a crown is, my staff will say, "A crown can cost anywhere from $400 to $1200, depending on what needs to done and what insurance coverage you have." They immediately then take control of the call, because if they wait, the caller is going to ask another price question.

If a caller asks how much a root canal costs, my staff would say, "A root canal can be anywhere from $500 to $1200 depending on what tooth it is and how many canals are inside." A good way to get price shoppers into the office is offer a free consultation.

Sit down with your team and decide what ranges you want them to give out for different procedures when patients call and ask. If you don't discuss this with your team, they will always produce that *verbal vomit* that kills the case.

Any patient question, no matter what it is, is really just asking,

"Is your dental office right for me?" Answer the questions as best as you can, but always with the attitude that you want to convey to them that your office is a great place to be.

Anatomy of a Call: Same Day "Emergencies"

I put the word "emergencies" in quotes because what we feel is an emergency is often very different from what a patient feels is an emergency. You must realize that if the patient feels they have an emergency, you need to find a way to see them that day, or at least first thing the next morning.

Your team needs to understand that if the patient is sounding like they want something looked at, no matter how trivial it *really is*, it needs to be looked at as soon as possible.

Anytime a parent calls about a concern over something with a child, they need to be seen. Even if they are calling because the lower permanent centrals are coming in lingual to O and P, I assure you that this is an emergency in the parent's eyes. Essentially, any problem-focused call involving a child is an emergency to the parent.

If a patient is having post-operative sensitivity, your staff can explain that it sounds pretty normal, but they need to offer to have the patient seen by the doctor that day if the patient wants to. Usually the patient just wants the reassurance that what they are feeling is normal, but if you don't offer to see them and they wanted to be seen, they will feel as if you dismissed their concerns as not important. When patients feel dismissed, they often dismiss themselves from your practice.

All in all, if patients want to be seen, they need to be seen. If you don't, you will lose that patient to the next office they call that will see them that day. We have acquired many new patients because their existing office couldn't look at them that day. If you can't see same day emergencies, some other dentist will, and you can consider those patients as good as gone.

No Second Chances to Make a First Impression

The phone is the first interpersonal contact the patient will have with your office. It's one of the earliest touch points in the *dental sales process*. You only get one chance to make it great and set the tone for the rest of the relationship you will have with that patient. The entire team needs to have phone training, even the clinical staff. You never know who is going to answer the phone. I am confident that anyone at my office can effectively handle the phone and convert new patients. Make sure everyone is trained so that a great first impression is always made when a new patient calls.

Confirmation Calls

While you should be using an automated text and email platform to confirm the majority of your appointments, you will have to call some people each day. Your wording is important. I hear a lot of offices say things like, "Hi, this is so and so from the dental office calling to confirm your appointment tomorrow at 9 AM. If you can't make it or need to reschedule, please call us at 555-5555." What that really says to the patient is that it's OK to cancel. I don't want my patients to ever think they can cancel on me. If they do, we always schedule them out at least a month or two. We need to train our patients that our time is valuable and must be taken seriously.

A better way to do a confirmation is to say, "Hi John, this is _____ from Nelson Ridge Family Dental and I was calling to remind you of your appointment tomorrow at 9AM. We have this time reserved only for you and look forward to seeing you tomorrow!" It sounds a lot different than the previous example, doesn't it? Give that script a try. Never express to the patient that it is ok to cancel, because if you do, they will as soon as something better to do comes along. Do you think your patients could find something more fun to do than go to the dentist? You bet!

Dealing with Answering Machine Cancellations

One thing that will dramatically decrease your cancellations over the answering machine during after hours is adding this simple phrase to the end of the message:

"Please note that we cannot accept cancellations through voice mail and that late cancellations will be assessed a $75 charge."

I don't ever want you to charge anyone should they cancel via the answering machine, but I assure it will make some people think twice before they do. Try it and see.

Hold It Right There

In a perfect world, your office would only get one call at a time. We all know what the reality is. At some point, a patient will need to be placed on hold. Being placed on hold is very common in dealing with businesses and it can be done considerately.

First, **slow down**. Often when we are going to place someone on hold, we talk very fast, because we may be in a hurry to get to another call or task. Anytime you place someone on hold, **ask for permission**. The patient will always answer yes. You must, however, wait for their response. Asking to place someone on hold and then hitting the button before they answer is very rude. Make sure you wait to hear their response.

Once they respond, **thank them** and hit the hold button.

Remember, we are a grateful and appreciative practice. Once you come back on the line, **thank them** again for holding.

Smooth Transfers

Whenever you are transferring a call to another team member, make sure you tell the caller why, tell them whom you are transferring them to, and ask permission. An example would be, "Mrs. Jones, I am going to transfer you to _____ so that she can answer all of your questions about your statement, is that ok?"

Insurance Talk

Dentists always complain about the pains of dealing with insurance. It would be nice if all our patients were cash only, and had the cash to pay for all recommended treatment. In reality, insurance is often a primary determining factor when patients are selecting a dentist. If we immediately jump into insurance questions when we take a new patient call, we are making it a primary factor on our end as well.

Insurance discussions should always come last. That's right, after all of the previous elements. This can be a difficult habit to retrain, but it is essential, especially when dealing with out of network patients.

Build value during the beginning portion of the new patient call, so that insurance coverage becomes less of an issue at the end.

Audits Build Excellence

As I said before, if you don't audit it, chances are it won't be done the way you want. Once you know how to convey to your team how you want the phone answered, you can then listen and evaluate their calls. Our evaluation sheet is shown below.

Homework

Work on those phone skills! Is there a standard format your staff works off of to encourage patients to make appointments? Most offices haven't bothered to formalize their phone system. It's time to start. Use the Anatomy of a Call section and write your own format for staff. Then have a meeting with your front desk team, and refine it. Explain the principles of ethical persuasion and work together to create a format that gets callers to book those appointments.

PHONE CALL EVALUATION SHEET

Employee name _____

Call date time _____

Mark 0 for does not meet expectations
Mark 1 for meet expectations
Mark 2 for meet expectations

GENERAL ELEMENTS	SCORE	COMMENTS
Greetings Script		
Thanks caller		
Gets name of caller		
Uses name		
Pace of speech		
Takes control of call		
Empathy/Value/Hope Statement		
Asks for appointment		
Uses alternatives		
Sets expectations for visit		
Promotes Doctor/Practice		
Insurance last		
HOLDING/TRANSFERRING		
Asks permission for hold		
Waits for response		
Thanks caller for holding		
Tell caller why and whom transferring		
Asks permission		
GENERAL PROFESSIONALISM		
Friendly		
Enthusiastic		
Sincere		

Total Score _____ (average of numbers)

Evaluator _____

CHAPTER 11
THE TRUE TEST—IN-OFFICE PX

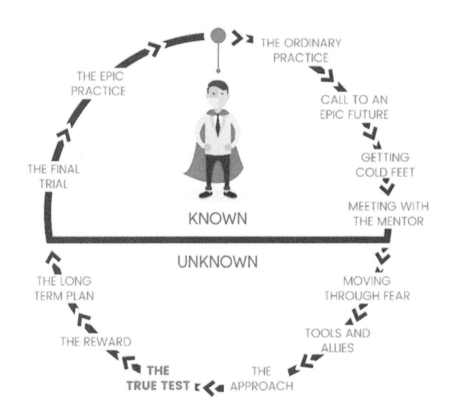

THE ORDINARY
PRACTICE

THE EPIC
PRACTICE

CALL TO AN
EPIC FUTURE

GETTING
COLD FEET

THE FINAL
TRIAL

MEETING WITH
THE MENTOR

KNOWN

UNKNOWN

THE LONG
TERM PLAN

MOVING
THROUGH FEAR

THE REWARD

TOOLS AND
ALLIES

**THE
TRUE TEST**

THE
APPROACH

It's time to take the leap, wield your weapon, and command your team. We've reached the heart of the maze. This is the monster you need to conquer, the beast that will provide the key to everything you've ever dreamed of. It's time to grapple with your in-office Patient Experience. Are you hero enough to take on the challenge?

In-Office PX is the Silver Bullet

What can excellent in-office PX do for you? It will decrease the number of people leaving your practice, will increase your case acceptance, and increase your word of mouth referrals.

Every touch point is important, and all of them are part of the new patient experience. If a touch point goes badly, it will destroy the work you've already done. Remember our balance scale? Off-brand touch points have much more weight than on-brand ones.

Think of it as a graph as the patient moves through your office. Every touch point builds off another. And in the end what your patient does is the sum of how well you execute each touch point in a positive and on-brand manner.

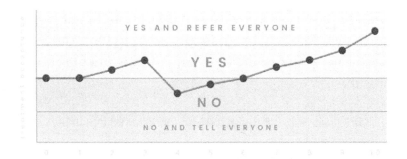

If you have enough positives, the patient will say yes. If you have even more, they will say yes and refer some of their friends and family. If you have enough negatives, the patient will say no and break up with you nicely. Patients do this by saying, "Uhhh...I have to check my schedule, I'll get back to you." Not every patient that says that is really breaking up with you, but that's how most of them do it when they do. If you have a lot of negatives or just one big one, the patient will say no, as well as tell everyone on social media and the internet how much your office sucks.

Many people have had absolutely horrible dental experiences in the past. We want to create an experience that is so different from their past ones that they will be almost speechless. We do that by being very specific about how the patient is going to move through and experience our office. We do that by creating a **movement sequence**.

Let's Move

A movement sequence describes how patients move through your practice. This is how you get consistency and make sure that all of the "little things" happen that make a big impression on your patients. A good sequence to start at is the new patient sequence. Sit down with your team and decide what you want to happen every time a new patient comes to your office. For instance, in my practice the new patient movement sequence goes like this:

Waiting Room (This sets the entire tone for the patient's first impression.)

1. The front desk person stands, smiles, and greets the new patient to welcome them to the practice.
2. They address the patient by name and welcome them to the practice.

3.   They ask for the ID and insurance card.

4.   They give the new patient paperwork to the patient.

5.   They point out the coffee bar and fridge and ask the patient to "make themselves at home."

6.   They point out the restrooms, so that the patient can find them easily.

7.   After the patient returns the paperwork, the receptionist thanks them and tells them that she is letting the people in the back know that they are ready to be seated.

8.   Person from the back comes to get patient.

Clinical Staff (Assistant/Hygienist)

1.   Smiling, they walk into waiting room and approach the new patient.

2.   They address the patient by the age appropriate name.

3.   They invite the patient to follow them to the back.

4.   If the patient is a child, they ask the parent if they'd like to come back and if they have any questions or concerns for the doctor.

5.   They lead the patient to the operatory and make small talk.

6.   They offer to take the patient's coat and other belongings, hang up coats, and put belongings on the ottoman.

7.   They place the patient's bib.

8.   They explain what will be done today, and ask if there are any questions.

9.   They begin the new patient interview.

10. They begin the appointment and ask questions to get to know the patient on a personal level.

11. They obtain all necessary diagnostics.

12. They discuss any recommended or elective treatments.

13. They page the doctor.

14. They set the patient chair to preset #1, upright and elevated.

15. They brief the doctor outside the room, if possible.

Doctor Entrance

1. When the doctor enters, the hygienist turns the TV input to "Computer" so that there is no sound or movement on the screen.

2. The doctor sits in the doctor chair with chart and makes small talk to develop rapport.

3. "OK, <Hygienist name>, what have we got?" is a handoff back to hygiene.

4. The hygienist walks in front of the patient and faces both the doctor and the patient while she briefs the doctor on the case.

5. The doctor asks any relevant questions before going through X-rays.

6. The doctor examines the x-rays with the patient, pointing out pertinent details.

7. The doctor asks permission to lean the patient back and leans them back.

8. The doctor examines the teeth and formulates a treatment plan, if possible.

9. The doctor returns the patient to preset #1 (upright, elevated) and places himself in front of the patient.

10. The doctor presents a treatment plan, using radiographs and other visual aids.

11. The doctor asks open-ended questions to gauge how the patient feels about the diagnosis and treatment and to spot any misunderstandings or objections.

12.   The doctor explains to the patient that the treatment coordinator will take over from here, and hands them off to the treatment coordinator.

Remember that you can always add to the sequence later as you think of things to make the new patient experience better. It's important that you start by getting clear on what you and your team want the patient to experience and how they logistically move through the office.

Notice how detailed our experience is when the patient arrives. Now that it's in writing, and the whole team has agreed on it, it's very clear what the expectations are for the team in how they handle the new patients. If you don't discuss these things with your team, every member will do it differently. Some will be better than others and some will do very poorly. You want consistency, so you need to be clear about what happens at your practice.

It's especially important to detail when and where hand-offs occur between team members. These are the places where it's easy to "drop the baton" and ruin the patient experience. Hand-offs allow you to reinforce your findings and recommendations with the patient as well as ensure that everyone who has "custody" of the patient knows what is going on.

You can make a movement sequence for pretty much any procedure or patient appointment. Once you start thinking about these, you will start noticing where you need them. We have sequences for existing patient recalls, patient on doctor's side, orthodontic or cosmetic consults, SRP appointments, suture removals, financial presentations, and orthodontic checks. The new patient sequence is the most extensive, while the suture removals sequence is very basic. Make your sequences as detailed as you want, but don't over complicate them, or no one will read or follow the sequence.

All the Practice is a Stage

Always think about everything happening at your office as a play. Just as a play is designed to entertain and delight its audience, your patient experience should do the same. Every patient, every day, more or less experiences the same rehearsed and performed play provided by your team day in and day out. Your dialogues, your dental analogies, and your handoffs can all be discussed and rehearsed to find what works best for your patients' experience.

I have quite a few speeches when talking about certain things to patients that I am sure anyone on my staff could repeat verbatim. We are all like actors/actresses in a play, performing the same one over and over each day for different audiences.

I read a story about Donna Marie Asbury, an actress who has been playing the same character in the play "Chicago" for over 16 years! She has performed more than 6600 shows! She mentions in the article how she occasionally thinks she can't do it anymore, but as soon as the countdown to curtain comes, she gets excited and gives it her all.

We need to be like Asbury, giving it our all every time we see a patient. I have young daughters right now, and we are making our third trip to Disney soon. My oldest is excited to meet Moana from the recent Disney film. I promise you, I don't care what is going on in that actress's life when my daughter meets her, but I want her to give it her all and make that experience special for my little girl.

All of us have bad days at the office. At some point we all say that we don't think we can do this stuff anymore. That's part of being human. But your enthusiasm in carrying out your play to its fullest potential each day is what your patient not only wants, but needs, so that they can say yes to your recommendations.

Patients want to feel like you care about them, that they can trust you, that you want what's best for them, that you haven't been out all night drinking, that you got enough rest, that your marriage is strong and you are a good parent, that everything is perfect in your life and there isn't anything on your mind that could possibly take your concentration off them. They want to believe that they are the center of your world, that you were born to serve them, that you are going to be available when they need you, and most of all, that you are and will continue to be the best dentist in the world.

I know it's unrealistic, but sit down and think about that some time. Orchestrate your play to be the dentist *they* want you to be.

Brand Standards are the Best Standards

Every business has non-negotiables for their product called the Standards of Service. Just as we have clinical standards of care, such as you wouldn't remove a wisdom tooth without an X-ray, we can have standards for in-office patient experience. Again, these are non-negotiable, meaning they happen every time, for every patient.

For example, at my office we have decided that when patients enter our practice, the person at the front will always acknowledge them immediately. If they are available, this is an enthusiastic greeting. If they are on the phone, it's a quick gesture, like smiling, waving hello, and then mouthing, "I'll be with you in one second," or whispering to the patient, "Have a seat and I'll be with you in a moment," while covering the mouthpiece on the phone.

Our standard is that the patient *must* be acknowledged. I remember when I went to a certain doctor's office for the first time. I stood at the window while two women were on the phone with their heads down and another towards the back was making copies of some records or something. None of them acknowledged me. I eventually sat down and waited for about ten minutes before getting up again. They still hadn't acknowledged me even though they were now off the phone. I walked back up to the window, and said "Hello." One of them looked up and asked my name and then told me I was ten minutes late. I was furious. I never went back there again. Do you think that office sets their standards of service? No, they don't.

Another example is that after every restorative appointment, a patient will receive a warm towel before getting up and being escorted out. This happens every time. If it doesn't happen every time, it's inconsistent, and our patients crave consistency. This consistency is a big part of our brand identity. The standards for patient experience reinforce our brand.

I've heard an anecdote about someone who went to a barber shop and had his hair scissor-trimmed on the sides. He was really happy with his experience at the shop and his haircut. He returned to the same barber shop in a month for another cut. This time, the same barber used the clippers to trim the sides of his hair instead of the scissors. The customer was a little bummed, as he really liked the scissor-only look. The customer decided to give it a third try a month later; this time it was a scissor trim followed by some of the electric clippers. After the third inconsistency, the customer no longer felt as positively about the barber shop.

Our patients want to know that what they came to the office and received last time will be consistently available the next time, and to anyone they refer to our office. Consistency is key. Consumers make the decision of what level of quality they want before they leave their house. They then go to the place that can most consistently deliver that level of quality. You need to be that place!

No One Remembers the Middle

Hermann Ebbinghaus was a 19th century German who noticed that people often remember the first item and the last item in any sequence. He termed his finding the Serial Position Effect. I like to think of every interaction with a patient like that. I want to start it well and end it well.

If I am in a big hurry trying to get caught up, I might step on the gas a little while drilling and filling, but when I walk into the room, I am calm and talk slowly. I enthusiastically greet the patient and make a little small talk. Also, when I sit the patient up after the procedure is completed, I mentally make myself slow down and give them a proper post op instruction experience. I always let the patient know that if they need anything, they should call me, even if it's on a weekend. I thank them, tell them it was good to see them, and touch them on the shoulder as I walk out. That's how you end well. If I can start and end well, I feel like the patient will forget about any sense of urgency they picked up from me while I was working. They'll just think, "Man, that guy was fast!"

Better Acting Through Body Language

If the practice is a stage, and we're putting on plays for our patients, body language matters. When you're watching a play, the actor's facial expressions and movements convey almost as much meaning as the words. That's why Shakespeare often makes more sense on stage than it does when you read it. Fine-tune your body language to give your patients a great patient experience.

You're Never Fully Dressed without a Smile

The easiest way to make patients feel good is to smile. Smiling says, "I am not judging you," or "I have judged you positively."

Do you know anyone who is always smiling? They are likeable people. They make the people around them feel good. Every interaction should begin and end with you smiling. I don't care if you have to fake it; start being a dentist that people enjoy being around.

Posture Speaks Louder than Words

What does a confident person look like? How about a depressed person Think about their posture. The confident person will be standing or sitting up straight, and the depressed will be slouching.

Your patients want to sense your confidence. Make sure your posture is in alignment with what you are trying to portray. I once heard a podcast in which an entrepreneur named Jordan Harbinger of the Art of Charm explained how once you are interacting, your body language is a key part of the experience for the listener. You need to sit or stand up straight. But if you focus on your body language, you won't really connect, as your mind will be distracted. That's why he recommended doing what he called the doorway drill. Every time you walk through a door, you remind yourself to stand up straight and put your shoulders back. That way you condition your body to stand up straight all the time. Once you are interacting with someone, hopefully you keep this posture without thinking about it, and they perceive you as confident and comfortable.

The body never lies. Ask you team what your body language says. Be comfortable enough in your own skin to take some criticisms from them. You know what kind of things you want to represent. Ask your team how you can improve.

I remember where for a week or two I would start turning the doctor chair around backwards and sit facing the patient like some kind of cool 90's movie heartthrob. I was comfortable and relaxed. My hygienists called me out on it immediately;

they said it was awkward and strange. Those really weren't the adjectives I was going for. Had they not told me, I would still be doing it, being as "cool" as ever (at least in my own mind).

Homework

Sit down with your team and create a new patient movement sequence. Get clear on what things need to happen at each touch point to reinforce your brand and provide a great patient experience.

CHAPTER 12
THE TRUE TEST—THE WEIGHT OF THE WAITING ROOM

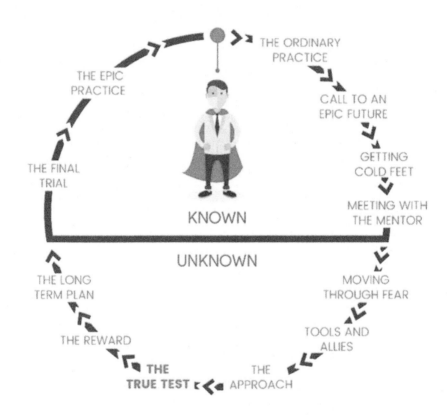

Just like the touch points on the phone before the patient arrives, there are a set of things that need to happen once the patient is in our waiting room. These are the non-negotiable standards of service I discussed in the last chapter. They need to happen every time so that your practice is consistent. When patients know that we will consistently take great care of them, they can confidently refer friends and family to us, knowing we will provide the same experience to them.

Greetings, Human

When the patient arrives, they need to be greeted warmly by name and with a smile. There are three elements there: warmly, by name, and with a smile. All three things need to happen. Your front desk person needs to be someone who is very outgoing and friendly. Do not put the shy person at the front. The receptionist is one of the most critical players on your team, and they need to be special.

How do you know the patient's name when you have never met them before? You make an educated guess. First you need to start a system of getting a picture of all your patients. Most practice management systems allow a patient picture in the chart. I have found the least awkward way to get this picture is to scan their driver's license picture. Tell the patient you need it for insurance verification. Scan it and crop the picture out.

Now that you have pictures of your existing patients, you can look at the schedule and see who is coming around the same time as a new patient. There are likely at most three or four people coming in around that appointment time.

Since you are going to recognize the people that have already been at the office, you now know that if you don't recognize that person, they are likely the new patient. You need to say, "Hi, Mrs. Smith, welcome to the practice! We are very happy to have you!" That will make a great first impression!

What if they are not Mrs. Smith? What if you have two new patients coming at the same time? What if Mrs. Jones was also a new patient and coming in at the same time as Mrs. Smith? If you call Mrs. Jones the wrong name, she will let you know, and then you can say, "Well then, you must be Mrs. Jones!" The patient will not be upset if you get it wrong the first time meeting them and honestly, it won't happen very often.

Another reason to review the pictures of the patients on the schedule is so that you can greet your existing patients by name. This will go a long way to making your patients feel welcome in your practice. They are our guests, and we want them to feel at home.

An important aspect of the greeting is being professional. While the younger generations may feel it is ok to call people older than them by their first names, a lot of the older folk will appreciate you calling them Mister, Misses, Sir, or Ma'am. My rule of thumb is that if the person is ten years older than you, they are mister or misses. If the patient says you can call them by their first name, then you have permission. If you want to stay on the safe side though, always call patients by their last name and the appropriate title, especially with the older generation. When patients do give me permission to use their first names, I always say, "I'll try, but I may call you Mr. Jones out of respect, because that's how I was raised."

A Sense of Direction

After the greeting, tell the patient what you need them to do and make them feel at home. Gather any insurance cards or identification that you need from the patient and then hand them the new patient paperwork and tell them to have a seat and bring it back to you when you are done. Let them know that if they need any help, you would be glad to help them.

Next we need the **good host statement**. A waiting room should look like a comfortable home. By the same token, I want to treat the patient like a guest in our home. We do this by offering our good host statement.

In my practice, we have a fridge full of bottled water and a Keurig coffee maker. Our patient bathroom is past the door separating the clinic area from the waiting room. I want the patient to know what is acceptable for them to do while they wait. If you don't tell them, they will be unsure.

My front desk person will say to them, "There is bottled water in the fridge if you would like some. There is also a coffee maker if you would like to brew a cup. If you need to use the washroom, it's straight through that door right there." Now the patient knows that they can take some water, make some coffee, or use the washroom without asking.

I have a friend who has cake in his waiting room every day. When he started this, he noticed that the cake often went uneaten. He then had his front desk person start telling the patients to have a slice of cake if they wanted. Guess how much cake started getting eaten? You guessed it! A whole bunch! If you are going to offer treats to your patients, make sure you verbally offer it to them. This will go a long way to making your patients feel special and at home in your practice.

Who Sent You?

As far as I am concerned, I have two types of "Very Important Patients": those patients that refer other people to us, and the people that they refer. These are the most valuable patients you have. Only a small percentage of your patient base will refer a large number of patients to the office. These are the people that somehow find a way to talk about you when they are out at social gatherings, no matter what the conversation is about. Other patients may refer someone if prompted by a friend to make a recommendation, but they will not go out of their way to refer people like your VIPs.

When a new patient checks in, I want to know how they heard about us before they come back. If they came from an existing patient referral source, I want to know who that is, so that I can talk to the patient about how much I like that person. The more important reason why I want to know is that I want to really wow this new patient so that they can go back to their friend and tell them what a great experience they received from the recommendation. It's so important that they have a great experience, because if they go back to the referral source and tell them that they weren't impressed, that source is now less likely to refer additional people to us. On the other hand, if the referral goes back to the source to thank them and say what a wonderful experience they had, that person is now much more likely to continue to refer more people to the practice. There are only two types of patients: those who refer and those who don't. We don't want to turn one that refers into one that does not.

Honestly, I try to treat everyone like VIPs, but if it is an existing patient referral, I will go that extra mile and spend a little more time with them. The other reason we always want to know the referral source is so that we can keep track of what marketing is working. This will help us see if we are getting any return on investment if we decide to run a newspaper ad or Facebook campaign.

At the end of the month, print out your new patient referral report and send each person on there a handwritten note thanking them for the referral. This note needs to be handwritten. If you are too busy, Doctor, then have someone on the staff be responsible for it. I used to write these myself, but now the team does it. Also, in the card, include a gift. This can be a $5 gift card for coffee, two free movie tickets, a $10 gift card to a restaurant, etc. If you call, most businesses would be happy to give you these for free or at a discount just to get the new business. Call around and see what you can find. You can change these up so that repeat referral sources never know what they are going to get.

There's No Waiting in the Waiting Room

My practice is an "on time practice." This is something I constantly stress to the team. We can run behind just like any other practice, but we always try to get the patient at least seated on time. If I am busy in another room, one of my hygienists will numb the patient for me, and the assistant will usually sit and chat with the patient if there aren't any preliminary impressions or informed consents to go over.

It's important that we understand the psychology of waiting. Psychologist David H. Maister produced the seminal report on the psychology of waiting in lines. He asserts that the quality perceived from a service organization can be affected by waiting times. So improving on this aspect of your practice will also improve how the patient perceives the quality you deliver. He continues to explain that there is a halo effect created by the early stage of any service encounter, meaning that if an experience starts positive, it has the most potential to stay that way. On the other hand, if we upset the patient by making them wait very long to be seated, it may be hard to recover from the ill feelings already created. So that if you want the biggest bang for your buck, pay attention to the earliest stages of any appointment. Maister outlined seven principles of waiting, which we'll review.

Principle 1 – Occupied time feels shorter than unoccupied time

The philosopher William James observed, "Boredom results from being attentive to the passage of time itself." This is why restaurants often hand out menus to parties that are waiting to be sat.

In this day in age, it's not hard to entertain in the waiting room. In our waiting room, we have a television that the patient can change to whatever they like, another television showing pictures of the team as well as before and afters, magazines, a book full of more before and afters, a computer hooked up to the internet, a beverage bar, and free wifi. It doesn't take a lot of thought to add something to your waiting room other than magazines. Get creative.

Principle 2 – People want to get started

People want to begin. That is another reason why handing out menus at the restaurant waiting area is effective. I like to apply this to the dental office by getting the patient back as soon as possible. That way we can get the forms signed, get some topical anesthetic going, get them numb, take any preliminary impressions and photos, etc. Once the patient is in the back and we are beginning to do things with them, they are no longer waiting. Sometimes, we just need to get them back and stall. Always get the patient into the room as soon as possible.

Principle 3 – Anxiety makes the wait seem longer

People can be anxious about a lot of things. Do you think they are anxious about dentistry? You bet! There isn't a whole lot we can do to alleviate this other than starting the appointment quickly. People are going to be anxious at the dentist and waiting will intensify that anxiety. Have some compassion and get them going!

Principle 4 – Uncertain waits are longer than known, finite waits.

If a patient is five or ten minutes behind their appointment time and still sitting in the waiting room, they will begin to wonder whether or not you forgot about them. Then they will start to wonder if they should go back up to the desk to check. This will produce even more anxiety, and remember what we said about anxiety?

Always let your patients know how much longer they will be waiting. This will let the patient know that you know that they are there and it will give the patient a time frame in which they will have to wait. If you tell the patient in the waiting room, "The doctor is running a little behind, we will be with you shortly," the patient doesn't know exactly how long that is, and the waiting seems longer. If you tell that patient, "The doctor is running about fifteen minutes behind, we will get you back as soon as we can," then the patient has a time frame. Initially, they may be upset that they have to wait, but since you have given them a time frame, they can then relax and accept it, rather than go through the anxiety of the unknown.

Principle 5 – Unexplained waits are longer than explained waits

In his article, Maister explains, "Waiting in ignorance creates a feeling of powerlessness, which frequently results in visible irritation and rudeness on the part of the customers as they harass serving personnel in an attempt to reclaim their status as paying clients."

This means that if we tell our waiting patients why we are behind, it will reduce their anger and anxiety about waiting. However, letting them know you are behind because you are overbooked is not a good idea. If you are going to give them a reason, make sure it is a good one.

Every time you are late getting to a patient, you need to

apologize. This needs to come from the doctor as well as the staff. Patients will forgive you, but if you do it multiple times they will not. If your patients are consistently waiting because you are running behind, you need to take a good hard look at your scheduling. Nobody wants to go to an office that is always late.

Principle 6 – Unfair waits are longer than equitable waits

This principle speaks to the fact that nobody likes to be cut in front of in line. We often run into this when a patient arrives early for their appointment, yet two other people come in after them and are sat before them. It's usually because they were seeing the hygienist, but the first patient can perceive this as not being valued since they were waiting longer than the other two that walked in on time and were sat on time.

When patients arrive early at my office, the front will let them know that they are early and that she will check to see if the doctor can see them early. She will then ask us if we can see them. If we can, great. If not, she lets the patient know that the doctor is not available right now but is running right on schedule and will seat them at their appointment time, which is 12:30. This way, the patient is aware that they are early, and that we are keeping our end of the bargain, even though we would have been willing to see the patient early if the schedule permitted. Nothing is worse than a patient who arrives early expecting to be seen early. Telling them that we will sit them on time keeps them from being upset.

Principle 7 – The more valuable the service, the longer the customer will wait

This should be obvious, but people are willing to wait longer for things they value. If you provide fantastic customer service and occasionally the patient has to wait a little past their appointment time to be sat, most will be forgiving. However, if you are just an average office with an average culture of customer service, patients will seek out another average office if you make them wait multiple times. If patients value what you provide, they will wait longer.

I have heard from many patients who have scheduled an appointment that coincided with something else going on in their lives tell me that they cancelled the other thing, because they didn't want to reschedule their dental appointment. How cool is that? Nothing is more of a litmus test than when your patients cancel their other obligations to be with you. Be that office!

The easiest way to keep patients from being upset about waiting is to not make them wait in the first place. Stay on schedule. If you are running behind and know it, text or call the patient so that they can come twenty minutes later. Have good communication between your front and back so that the front desk knows if you are on schedule or not. Sometimes a patient would rather reschedule than be sat twenty minutes late. When that happens, it is a blessing, since it solves the immediate problem of running behind. But if you are chronically late, don't expect these tactics to keep your patients happy. Sooner or later they will get tired of you not valuing their time.

Homework

Get to the office early and sit in your waiting room for ½ hour. How do the chairs feel? Where do your eyes go? What is ugly? What is enjoyable? Sitting there, what do you wish you had?

Write down your impressions. Then write down one concrete thing that could improve your waiting room for patients.

CHAPTER 13
THE TRUE TEST—INTO THE OPERATORY

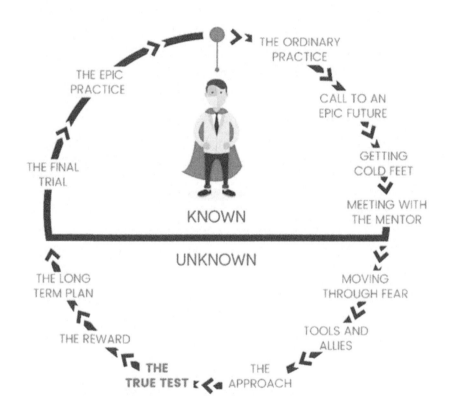

Your patient is frightened and uncomfortable. What you're about to say and do may cause them pain. Can you triumph and give them a heroically good patient experience anyway?

Once we get the patient into the operatory and get all of our diagnostics, we have to present our treatment suggestions. Whether or not they say yes to our treatment will largely be dependent on the patient-doctor interaction up to this point.

Every aspect of your interaction with that patient must be on -brand and positive, or they will never agree to treatment with you.

Establish Rapport the Moment You Walk In

People buy things from people they like. The patient needs to like you. The old adage that, "No one cares what you know until they know how much you care" applies in the operatory.

Getting to know your patients before you examine them will exponentially increase your case acceptance more than anything else.

Remember that doctor's office I went to, where the front desk people ignored me? Well, the doctor was pretty bad too. He walked in, didn't shake my hand or introduce himself, sat down, and said, "What is your pain?" I was really taken aback. It's amazing how much better of a job we can do when we look at people doing it very poorly. I did not leave with a good feeling about the doctor. He may have been the best in the world, but when dealing with patients, people skills and rapport go a lot further than credentials.

Before you start any sort of exam on the patient, you need to get to know them.

This is not an interview, it's a dialogue. You will make small talk, ask questions and hope you can take it somewhere relating back to you. That is how you make connections.

Always shoot for three connections before you start talking about teeth.

The internet has many resources on how to make small talk. I ask the same questions all the time to get the conversation going. I might be "profiling" a little here, but these are the questions I ask people depending on who is in the chair. Keep in my mind, my hygienists usually prepare me by giving me certain things to talk about, since they have already spent the past 40 minutes or so with the patient.

How to Talk to People in Their 20s

People in their 20s rarely have expendable cash, but they will do treatment if needed. Elective procedures are hard with this age group.

I ask:

- Where are you from?
- Are you in school or working?
- Where did you go to school?
- What are you studying? Or how do you like working there?

How to Talk to Men in Their 30s and 40s

An easy topic for most men is usually sports. Still, men place a lot of worth on what they do. It's what makes us men. But if I ask someone about their job and it seems like the patient doesn't want to talk about it, I move on to hobbies.

- What do you do?
- How long have you been doing that?
- Do you like it?
- Do you golf, fish, hunt, play sports, etc.

How to Talk to Women in Their 30s and 40s

Women often value their family and their kids. Almost always, we start talking about children. These are easy conversations.

- Do you have any kids?
- How old? Boys, girls?
- Who's watching them now? Are they at school?
- Do you think you may want to have more?

How to Talk to Men over 50

Men are easy because they can usually talk about their work. As they get older they might have kids transitioning into adulthood. Their kids might be getting married, graduating college, or even having babies and having their parents watch their grandkids a lot. Make sure to learn which of your patients follow which teams. Otherwise, you might praise the Cubs to a Sox fan and end up their least favorite dentist!

How to Talk to Women over 50

Women love to talk about their grandkids. Like *really* love to talk about them. Get them going; talk about your own kids. This is probably the easiest demographic to connect with.

- Do you have grandkids?
- Do they live close by?
- Do you see them a lot?

The main idea is to always link it back to yourself and find some common ground.

After I am done with getting to know the patient, I will turn to the hygienist and say, "Ok, <hygienist's name>, what do we got?" This is the hygienists cue to take over. Then the hygienist begins her briefing and we move on to the exam portion.

Always keep some kind of place in the chart for personal notes about the patient. This is how you develop relationships. We keep it on a hidden page in our PMS. The personal notes include things like what they do, info about their kids, any vacations coming up, etc. People are always impressed by how great my memory is. Good thing I don't run into patients too often outside of the practice, because I have one of the worst imaginable memories when it comes to people.

Common Pitfalls of Patient Experience

To create a great patient experience, you need to do things differently than most of our colleagues. Here are three things that doctors don't do that they should.

The Post-op Call

Every doctor hates them, but you need to make post op calls for any major procedure you do. I am not talking about fillings, but the big stuff like endo, extractions, cosmetics case, sedations, etc. Every time the phone is ringing, I pray that it goes to voice mail. Most of the time it does, because I call during the day. You just have to; it's part of the experience and will go a long way with your patients. If you can't make post-op calls, make sure you have someone on your staff who can do this.

Patients need follow-up to feel appreciated.

The Right Thing

We have a motto at my practice: "The patient is not always right, but it is our job to make them feel they are."

If a patient is upset about anything, make it right. If you quoted a copay incorrectly, make it right; don't blame the insurance company. If you don't want negative reviews, handle the upset patients in a way that makes them happy, even if you have to give them all of their money back.

I once wrote a patient a check for a $4000 implant-over-denture case, because the patient was having perio issues due to a lack of attached tissue around her mini-implants. I explained connective tissue grafting and such, but she just wasn't happy. I offered to remove the implants and give her all her money back. She was happy and I still see her and her entire family for care. You will never win by keeping an upset patient's money; the reputation damage and loss of patients will always cost more than the treatment you provided. Just give the refund.

You should always strive to handle conflict on-brand. I once ate at a fancy restaurant in Scottsdale and ordered a bone-in ribeye. It came almost 45 minutes later, was barely warm, and was the driest steak I have ever eaten. The waiter came back after delivering the food and said, "It was worth the wait, wasn't it?" I said, "Actually no, I hate to complain, but it's barely warm and really dry." He offered to remake it, but I didn't want to stick around and wait for it. He came back later and said, "We are going to comp your dessert since your steak was bad; here are the dessert menus." My wife and I rarely eat dessert and I said, "No thanks, we will just take the check." He said OK and walked away to get the check. I was now upset. I told my wife if he didn't comp that steak that I had two bites of, I was going to flip. I sat there and stewed about how I was going to leave one-star reviews on Google, Facebook, and Yelp. I was upset. The waiter came back with the check and, thankfully, had comped the steak. I was happy, I left a good tip, and I would return to that place. How different would it have been if he had charged me $70 for a steak I had two bites of? Always handle problems by making your customer happy. It will pay dividends down the line. Don't be short sighted and try to keep your money. It's never worth it, no matter how much in the right you are.

Set Lower Expectations

People often set expectations high to put the patients at ease. We will tell them a filling wasn't deep and they shouldn't have sensitivity. We tell them an extraction was easy, and it shouldn't be too sore later. We tell them that we are going to make them a great denture that they will be happy with.

Always explain to the patient the worst case scenario. For example, tell the patients that they will experience cold sensitivity for a month or so after a filling. Tell them that they will experience quite a bit of soreness or pain for a few days after a root canal. After placing an implant, tell them 10% of these will fail and we don't know why, but if it happens we will address it. Tell them how awful their immediate denture is going to be and that they probably won't eat anything with any sort of substance for a few months, if ever.

Set expectations low, then exceed them. It's not that hard. Howard Farran once said that he tells patients after they had a root canal to "get your gun out of your house when you get home, because when the anesthetic wears off, you are going to want to stick it in your mouth and blow your brains out!" If you know Howard, you probably believe he actually says that. How do you think his patient feels after they only have a little soreness that some ibuprofen can handle?

Patient Experience is the Biggest Differentiator

To distinguish yourself from corporate and the rest of the pack of dental offices, you need to be intentional about the things you do to enhance the patient experience. It's so easy to be different. All of the things presented in this chapter are not difficult to do. There is no reason why anyone shouldn't be able to improve their patient's experience and, in turn, their case acceptance by just tweaking a few things.

Homework

Google some articles on the art of small talk and building rapport. Commit to getting to know your next new patient as a person before you talk about anything dental with them. See if your treatment acceptance improves.

CHAPTER 14
THE TRUE TEST—TREATMENT PRESENTATION

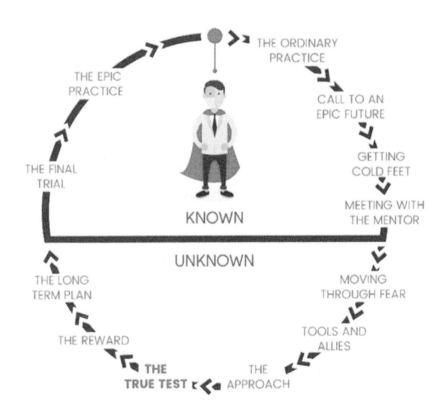

Treatment presentation is hard to learn and even harder to perfect. You have to be able to rely on your staff and your brand to help you convey treatment options to the patient. You simply want to do what's best for them and their oral health, but can you convince patients to accept your recommendations? If you can't master the art of treatment presentation, your practice will be doomed and you'll be a failed hero.

Treatment presentation isn't a matter of natural talent or luck. It's a skill that can be learned, practiced, critiqued, and improved. No one is perfect at it, and it's common to flub treatment presentations from time to time, especially early in your career.

Common Pitfalls

Here are some common pitfalls I see in many of my colleagues.

1. Overcomplicating

Dentists go through a lot of school. We learn a lot technical terms and the science to go along with it. However, most of our patients don't really care about technical details. In dental school, we were taught (incorrectly) that if we educated the patient, they would make the best decision. That couldn't be further from the truth.

I see most young dentists make the mistake of overcomplicating treatment by talking too much about details. I've heard this called the curse of knowledge—the more you know, the harder it is to explain.

You need to figure out an easy way to explain any treatment you provide. Your visuals and language need to be accessible to your patients. If you pay attention, you'll notice that when people don't understand what is getting explained to them, they shut down.

I hate when I get my oil changed and the guy brings me the oil filter to show me how dirty it is. Or when I get new tires and the guy is showing me some wear pattern on the brake pads or something. I don't know cars. They often try to explain it to me, but it rarely makes any sense. I often don't know whether to trust them or not, and it makes a buying decision hard, especially when they are talking about me spending more money than I had planned to.

I never want to seem like I don't know what they are talking about, so I just say, "Oh yeah, totally! I can see that. Yep!" And then when they ask me to replace something, I usually say, "I'm gonna think about it."

Your patients do the same thing. No one wants to seem unknowledgeable. Our intentions are always good when trying to educate the patient, but they often fail in what we are trying to do, which is lead them to a purchase.

I heard my associate go into a long diatribe about why a tooth needs a root canal. It was probably ten sentences or so. She then asked if the patient understood that. The patient said yes. Then she went into why a tooth with a root canal always needs a build up and a crown. It was a lot of information. It would have been easier to just say, "This tooth has a large cavity all the way into the nerve. If you want to keep this tooth and prevent a toothache, we will need to do a root canal, build up, and crown to fix it. Have you ever had a root canal?" Then answer any questions.

Think about what you are saying and how you can really shorten and dumb down the way you talk about procedures and recommendations. If you don't know how to present it, you might not even want to diagnose it sometimes. Hygienists are often guilty of this when they don't know how to present perio treatment.

Use visuals to show complicated things like why an implant is better than a bridge. Take pictures off the internet and save them on the computer so you can use them, or buy one of those models that show all the different possible restorations. You want to be able to have the patient understand the concepts without spending a lot of time talking about it. The more you talk, the more you confuse, and the more you confuse, the more likely the patient is to say, "I'm going to think about it."

2. Not Taking the Shot

A lot of dentists are afraid to ask patients about elective treatments. Wayne Gretzky said "You miss 100% of the shots you don't take." I have a personal vendetta against diastemas in the smile zone. I always ask the patient if they have ever considered closing that space between those two teeth. If they say yes, I will explain options. If they say no, I will just say, "OK, well if you ever think you may want to, let us know and I can explain a few different options for doing so." And then move on.

A lot of times, people will say no, but then right as I am about to leave the room they say, "If I wanted to close this space, what would you do?" They may also say no and then start to think about it more. They may begin to notice that their smile would look a lot better with the space closed. They might come back at their next appointment and ask about it. You never know.

Never judge whether a patient can afford big ticket treatment. You never know who can afford it and who cannot. Sometimes a big event is coming up in the patient's life and they are really motivated to get their smile redone. It can be a high school reunion, or even a divorce putting them back on the dating market. I have had patients say yes to big things right before a divorce, because they know everything they spend money on is 50% off since they are going to split all their debts with their spouse. You just never know. Take the shot and see what happens. It never hurts to ask and politely move on if they say no. You should always be planting seeds of what is possible.

3. Not Presenting Complete Treatment Plans

We can all agree that people dislike coming to the dentist. If you had somewhere you hated going, how much more would you hate it if each time you went, they told you that you needed to spend more money and time to fix things. And all the while, you are thinking, none of these things hurt.

Don't be a "watchodonist". If you see something that needs to be done, recommend it. I like to tell patients I don't care if we do it now or next year, but at some point we are going to have to address this. I plan large restorations for crowns on weakened teeth, because I don't like to watch them break. I hate when they break through the pulp and need endo or even worse, an extraction.

Why are we watching things we know need to be addressed now? Mostly because we don't want to be rejected and we are judging the patient as someone who will not want to have the treatment done. When we judge people as not being able to afford or want the dentistry, we are really just being selfish. We're not informing the patient on what we feel they should have done because we are insulating ourselves from rejection. You need to always take the shot and be consistent. Not only does it make your practice more productive, but it spares your patients pain and money in the long term.

My personal opinion on why a certain percentage of crowned teeth need endo eventually is because we wait until they break before we fix them. I may be wrong, but that is what I believe. I also believe in ethical dentistry and that you and I may not agree on what needs treatment. You have to do what is right in your own heart, but don't let fear of rejection keep you from presenting.

4. Using the Wrong Bait

What do fish like to eat? If they are really hungry, they will eat almost anything; but for the most part, fish like worms. If you want to catch fish, use worms.

Dentists often fail in treatment presentation by trying to sell the procedure instead of the benefits to the patient. A smile makeover should be so the patient can have more confidence and be more attractive, not so they have straight and white teeth. A tooth should be crowned to preserve the tooth long term so that they can eat whatever they want as they grow in old age and avoid a painful toothache, not because the tooth has had a lot of restorations and a direct filling would be unpredictable.

Patients want to know the benefits and how they relate to them. People want to be able to eat, avoid pain, and look younger. Sell the sizzle, not the steak.

5. Not Leading the Patient

Sales is really about leadership. It's leading the patient to a decision. Always tell the patient what you would do if it were your mouth. You can even tell them what work you, yourself, have had done. If you wouldn't do it in your own mouth, don't recommend it to the patient. You can never go wrong if you are honest.

Don't give the patient too many options. Keep it to one or two, or at most, three. If you are going to present options, always follow with what you would do. The more options you give, the more you will confuse, and we all know where that eventually goes.

I can't tell you how many times when talking to doctors I will just plain out ask them, what would you do if you were me? That's all I really care about. They are experienced professionals. If I trust them, I will do anything they recommend.

While we are talking about options, I want to mention two visuals I use at my practice. One is for implant overdentures and one for whitening. I made some visuals that only give three options. There are pictures I show on the computer screen and they allow me to easily explain what is possible.

When we used to sell whitening trays, people would always say, "$200? Wow, I'll just try some whitening strips first." Then we came up with a visual. We put the whitening trays, or "economy trays," at the left. The chairside "Boost" plus whitening trays are in the middle, and the "Max" is at the right.

I can tell you that in five years not a single person has done our "Max" option. It is really just two rounds of the middle option. The thing is, people rarely choose the most expensive option. Most choose the middle or the cheaper one. The great thing is that once they see that the most expensive is $700, the "economy" for $200 is not so bad.

I also do this with overdentures. I put mini implants on the left, a three implant overdenture in the middle, and a fixed hybrid on the right. In this case, for some reason, most people choose the middle option. Probably because I talk the mini implants down. Either way, I am happy placing implants under dentures any day of the week. Having a visual with limited options helps patients understand and move forward.

6. Not Walking the Patient Down the Stairs

I got this one from Dr. Chris Phelps. Always start with the expensive worse case scenario and then walk the patient down the stairs.

For example, if a tooth has a large filling or a fractured marginal ridge, explain to the patient that the tooth is weak and if you let it break, it could break through the nerve chamber and need a root canal, build up, and crown—which may cost in the ball park of $2500. Even worse, if it breaks down the root, we may need to remove it and replace it with an implant which could cost almost $4000. However, if we get a crown on it now, we can usually prevent the root canal and only spend around $1000, and your insurance may cover a portion of it too! Once they get the treatment plan and find out that their insurance covers half, they are feeling even better about it. The patient should feel pretty good about the crown at this point. Take them down the stairs, not up.

7. Not Talking about Advancements in Dentistry

Get excited about the advances in dentistry. Talk about the new porcelains, CBCT guided surgeries, advancements in implant dentistry etc. Don't get too detailed, but patients love to hear that you are passionate about what you do and you need to sell that sizzle. And let's be honest, it's cool stuff. Sometimes we forget how miraculous modern dentistry seems, because we work with it every day.

8. Not Asking Open-ended Questions

If you ever get the feeling that the patient is not on board or that you may have confused them, ask them something like, "Tell me what you are thinking now?" Or "Tell me how you are feeling about all of this?"

It's an awkward question usually, but just wait for a response. The patient will give you an answer that clues you into what might be keeping them from proceeding or what they are confused about. They may say, "I know I need it; I am just worried about how much it is going to cost." You can then explain that your treatment coordinator will go over all the fees and discuss financing if they should need it. By asking an open-ended question, you get to see what their objection, if any, might be.

If you just ask, "Do you have any questions?", you may not get that information. The patient will usually just say, "No."

9. Being Condescending or Rude to their Staff

Have you ever been around a couple that bickers at each other, or a person that constantly complains about their spouse when their spouse is standing right next to them? It's uncomfortable to be around. The people who usually do this think it is funny and cute, but in reality it makes everyone in the room feel uneasy.

Say please, say thank you. Be polite to your staff. Everyone knows you went to more school than them; it never gives you the right to be a jerk. Always tell the patient how great your staff is. If you are going to hand them off to the treatment coordinator, tell the patient that your treatment coordinator is the best and she is going to take great care of them. If a patient is being planned for SRP's, tell them that their hygienist is the best in the practice and is who cleans your teeth. I tell the patients all the time who the best hygienist in my practice is. It's always the hygienist they are going to see!

10. Not Understanding that Treatment Rejection is not a Rejection of You

I know what you are thinking: "Treatment acceptance is paramount to a successful practice!" It is, and your job is to create the value in your treatment so that patients want to follow through. In the end though, you cannot hold everyone's hand through the treatment process. You can't pick them up at their house, organize their finances so that they can afford treatment, or guarantee that their anxiety about treatment won't get the best of them. It's just not your problem!

One of my greatest mentors is Bruce Baird of the Productive Dentist Academy. I put my own take on his work, so I apologize if it isn't exactly what he teaches. You need to realize that although you want what is best for your patients' dental health, it's not always what they want. It could be finances, fear, or just plain not caring about their teeth. But guess what—*that's not your problem, it's the patient's!* If the patient doesn't follow through on what you recommend, it will lead to more dental work, and once they are in pain, they will be back. Even then, *it's still not your problem, it's the patient's!*

So what exactly is your problem? Your problem is to accurately and ethically diagnose and present recommended treatment to the patient, and then explain the risks if they don't follow through. You should also explain options if need be. That's it.

It's important that the entire team understands their role as health care practitioners. They need to help the patient realize the etiology of their disease and that they are in control of their dental health. We do this easily by educating the patient.

Educate, Educate, Educate

This is the foundation of my practice philosophy when it comes to recommending treatment. As I see it, there are only three ways we lose teeth: caries, periodontal disease, and mechanical factors.

If we can control all the risk factors for these three areas, there isn't any reason why our dentistry shouldn't last a long time. We need to communicate this philosophy to the patient. If we recommend something and they don't control their risk factors, it is now their problem when things fail.

Explaining Caries

To explain caries, I tell patients that cavities are caused by acid which is introduced into our mouth by our diet as well as by the bacteria in our mouths that break down the food we eat and the things we drink. I tell them that saliva buffers the acid, but takes around 30 minutes to bring the pH of the mouth back to neutral. If we constantly drink acidic or sugary drinks, we are always acidic, and the good bacteria can't live in that environment. They die off and the bad bacteria that love acid then overpopulate. This causes more cavities which then become a home for more bad bacteria. They then start producing enormous amounts of acid to the point where it doesn't matter if we stop drinking sugary and acidic drinks and brush our teeth 20 times a day, because the acid that the bad bacteria produce will inevitably keep our mouths acidic. This is how cavities snowball quickly once there are large areas of decay in the mouth.

I then explain that this is the reason that a lot of people "always have had bad teeth." I roll this into why it is important to do complete caries control in order to return to a baseline pH in which normal bacterial balance is achieved.

Most importantly, I tell the patient that no matter what we do, if they don't do complete caries control, the cavities will always spread to neighboring teeth and we will be fixing things every year. Also, if they continue their diet, nothing is going to work, no matter how good the dentistry. The blame is now on the patient, and they have a good reason to do comprehensive treatment. They take ownership over their disease because they now understand that it is *their problem!*

Explaining Periodontal Disease

Mostly, my hygienists do the education about periodontal disease. I just walk in the room and say, while looking at their x-rays, "I know that <Hygienist> already explained the condition of your gums in detail, so I won't spend any more time on it unless you have questions." I briefly point out the bone loss and calculus, and then move on.

If I were to explain it, I would say that there are pockets of tissue around the teeth that harbor bad bacteria. I say that these bacteria leak toxins into the bone and into the blood stream, which affects our systemic health and causes the bone to melt away. I like to add that there is often no pain associated with the disease until it is close to the point of removing all your teeth and getting dentures.

Lastly, I tell the patient that they need to have the bacteria removed by gum therapy, and that they will need to clean their teeth more than twice a year for the rest of their life. I want them to understand that if they don't come in for periodontal recare, they will eventually lose their teeth and continue to have these toxins and bacteria in their blood streams causing other systemic issues. I will explain the major risk factors such as smoking, diabetes, lack of flossing, and not getting their teeth cleaned.

What just happened? I explained to the patient that it was their risk factors that caused the disease, and that it is up to them to get their gums healthy and keep them that way.

If they don't follow through with treatment and proper recare, then they know it's *their problem!*

Explaining Mechanical Factors

This is comprised of two areas: overfunction and weakened teeth. By overfunction I mean bruxism, chewing ice, or any other habits that destroy teeth. By weakened teeth I am talking about teeth with large fillings or fractures.

I like to explain that no matter what dentistry we do, it will always fail if we don't control bruxism. Patients always want to balk at the idea of paying for a night appliance if their insurance doesn't cover it. That's ok, as long as they understand that things will break and it's because of their nighttime habits. After all, it's *their problem* not mine.

I use the intraoral camera to show them large fillings and fractures in teeth. I don't believe that we should wait for teeth to break. We can prevent that by protecting restored teeth with porcelain. I always let the patients know that we never know when they are going to break. It could be tonight, it could be in five years; but when it does, there is a chance that a tooth could need a root canal or need to be removed, if it doesn't break favorably.

I like to let them know that if they choose to not follow through with recommended treatment, that we will not badger them each time they come in for recare. I tell them that some people want to be proactive and others want to wait until things break and roll the dice. I respect either decision, because I really don't care either way. It's *not my problem!*

Please note that I never tell the patients, "It's not my problem." I just think that way. The greatest part about this is that it takes the patients' buying decisions off of our conscience. We did our part by diagnosing and informing and it doesn't have to matter to us whether or not they did theirs.

Education Helps Patients Understand Risk

Our goal should be to use these risk factors as a basis for treatment planning and educating the patient. We use these to sell our services and it is very persuasive.

If you explain risk factors to patients, they will often tell you that it makes so much sense, they can't believe no one has ever explained that to them before. It makes your exam different. It makes your treatment acceptance go up, and it shows the patient that you are really just looking out for them, not trying to make money to pay for your boat.

Give the Patient a Chance to be Ready

When treatment planning large elective treatments like cosmetics, orthodontics, or implants, always take the soft sell position. There are two types of selling, soft and hard. Hard sales are the ones used by people who work on commission. Think about when you are buying a car. The second that you express interest, they will not leave you alone. They will use closing sales tactics and be very high pressure. Nobody likes this sales approach. It causes us to put up our armor and shut down.

Soft selling is low pressure sales. You need to remember that a buying process grows longer as the price for treatment goes up. It is very unlikely to expect that you can get full commitment from the patient the day you first present a large treatment plan, especially for elective services. You really never know where they are in the buying process. It could be the first time they heard about veneers or even considered them. They may have heard of them but always thought they could never afford them. They may have researched it on the internet already or they may have not. You just never know.

I like to give "ballpark" figures when presenting large treatment. I think it is important to have the attitude that you will educate the patient and answer all his or her questions, but in the end, you aren't asking for a commitment at that visit. Always say something like, "Well, now you know about it and what it costs, so when you decide you are ready, you know where to find us." Or you can say, "We will be here when you are ready."

Communication specialist Paul Homoly talks about planting seeds for large treatment. You constantly plant seeds so that people eventually come back to you when they are ready. This can be next month, or five years from now. We don't know how long the patient will take to be ready, nor do we know if they ever will. All we can do is take a shot and present it.

If you hard sell someone and they buy from you, there will be buyer's remorse and the patient will not be happy. If the patient is truly ready, it's win-win on both sides. Have the attitude of, "when you are ready," because remember, whether or not they ever become ready is *not our problem*.

Homework

Great persuaders use scripts. To improve your case presentation, decide the best and most simple way to explain the need for a crown, a root canal, periodontal treatment, and a night guard.

Buy a wrist watch recorder and record your case presentation. Ask your hygienist or other team members to critique you. You can also record these on your phone. Don't worry about HIPPA. You are not sharing these with anyone and they likely won't have any personally identifiable information on them anyway.

CHAPTER 15
THE TRUE TEST—MONEY MATTERS

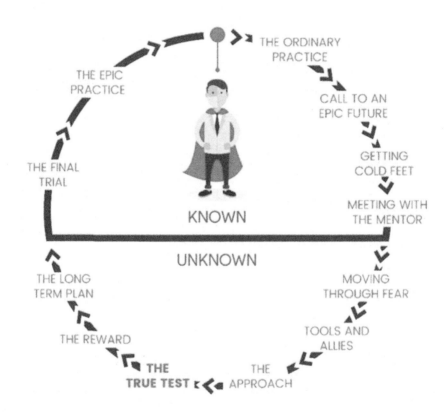

When a video game hero defeats a boss, the monster usually drops treasure. All the hero has to do is pick it up and warp home. When you're adventuring in the land of dentistry, it's not that easy. You can deliver the best patient experience in the waiting room and the operatory, but if you don't get a handle on your financial procedures, you'll still be hemorrhaging patients and cash. What's a dentist to do? As always, the answer lies in great systems run by great staff.

Fun with Financing

Our next set of systems has to deal with costs of treatment and making it easy for the patient to pay us for our services. This builds off the previous section of providing a great patient experience. We really don't have treatment acceptance until the patient's finances are completed and scheduled. We don't have true treatment acceptance until they show up for their appointment; but for all intents and purposes, treatment acceptance is when the patient schedules.

While many doctors may think that if they only had a great treatment coordinator, all of their problems would go away, that's just not the case. The clinical staff and the doctor need to create the need for the dentistry in the patient's mind. No matter what happens in the consult room, if the patient does not believe they need the treatment, they won't get it done. The easiest sells are getting the patient out of pain, but in reality, most of the treatment we recommend is on teeth that do not currently hurt. The clinical staff needs to help the patient answer the question, "Do I want/need it?" The treatment coordinator needs to help the patient answer, "Can I afford it?" If they don't want it, it really doesn't matter if they can afford it or not. No one is going to fix a "problem" they don't think they have.

When we have good financial systems and get our teams trained on them, production is bound to increase. In the

following section I will highlight my financial systems that
have worked well at my practice.

You Need Accurate Insurance Breakdowns

In our ideal dental world, we wouldn't have to file for the
patient; they would pay us full fee at the time of scheduling,
and any discrepancies would be the patient's problem. We
don't live in that world. Insurance is complicated and painful,
and so patients expect you to deal with it, since you're the guy
who deals in complicated and painful things.

In my opinion, most unhappy patients usually stem from
financial issues. They're the cases where we did not know that
their insurance downgraded posterior composites to
amalgams, or we didn't know there was a missing tooth
clause. There are a million little insurance clauses that make a
big difference in your patient's copay. You need to do your
best to get a detailed insurance breakdown so that your
estimates are pretty much exact. This takes longer on the
phone but saves a lot of headache down the line.

You need to ask the insurance about every little clause and get
an accurate estimate. What if your estimate was wrong and the
insurance didn't pay? For example, what if the insurance
didn't feel that periodontal therapy was supported by the
amount of calculus on the bitewings? Guess whose problem
that is? It's yours! Make the patient pay what you said they
would have to pay. Go read some negative Google reviews on
dentists. They often are, "They told me I had to pay this, and
then came back after they did the work and said I had to pay
an additional X dollars!" It's not worth the hassle of a bad
review. We can afford to do free work occasionally. Happy
patients are more important.

I once had a patient I did four crowns on. My front office

didn't ask the insurance about waiting periods on crowns. Guess what? I lost about $2000 of insurance money. Yep. I wrote it off and told the patient that though it isn't our fault, it wasn't their fault either. This patient is still at my practice and eventually did another 14 crowns in the next few years. I lost $2000 at one point with her, but she came back later and spent fourteen thousand. I assure you that money would have been lost if I had made the patient pay what the insurance wouldn't because of the waiting period.

This may be a big paradigm shift for people, i.e. writing off money that we are owed. The solution to not writing off things is to get an accurate breakdown of their coverage in the first place so that the pretreatment estimate is correct. You can solve this by preauthorizing everything, but if you do that you will lose the momentum of the patient ready to enter treatment, because you'll have to wait weeks for the insurance company to review it. So, just get the most accurate breakdown possible, and then honor your signed treatment plan like a contract when it comes to your patient's out of pocket.

How Much is a Tooth Worth?

Do this exercise with your team. Ask them what amount of money they would trade their front tooth for if they could never replace it. Most people wouldn't trade it for any sum of money. It's priceless. Think of the many dental cripples we see in our practices and the way that unattractive and diseased teeth inhibit them from truly enjoying life. Dentistry is truly life changing. We have the opportunity to change people's appearance in such a way that the whole direction of their lives are changed. Never forget that. *What is the value of a tooth?*

Although it's an easy principle to see when we are talking about missing front teeth, it even works for the day to day dentistry we do.

For example, if we treat a patient's perio condition, you might say the benefit is that they get to keep their teeth their whole entire life and can eat the things they enjoy. I want you think about it another way. What if they are single, and they meet an attractive person at the grocery store and eventually marry that person some years down the road—what would have happened if their breath was so repulsive from gum disease that they immediately turned the other person off? They would have never found love. The whole trajectory of their life would be different.

What about if we just treated someone with an occlusal filling? Pretty routine stuff, right? Well, imagine they let it go and eventually get a toothache and have to miss a day of work? What if that was the day something great was going to happen? What if they were going to meet the mate of their dreams like in the previous example? What if their boss was considering them for a promotion and that missed day was the turn off that caused the promotion to go to someone else? What if that occlusal decay eventually led to rampant decay some years later and the patient became a dental cripple? We see these things in our practice as small day to day procedures, but when you start thinking about the macro implications of not treating people, you can see how important dentistry really is. I know some of this may sound far reaching, but realize that it's all possible. We have an important job.

I do a lot of complete makeover charity cases, and I've seen that we have the power to completely change someone's life for the better. I also do quite a few rehabs where the patients are paying to get their smiles back. Most people don't even know what we are truly capable of. We can use our skills to improve people's lives. There is a lot of power in our hands.

Use it and appreciate it for what it really is.

So back to the example of the person who met his soul mate

and didn't scorch her face with his buzzard breath because his perio was treated. How much is that worth? I mean how much is it worth to land the woman of his dreams? Is it worth a cleaning that costs $1000? You bet; it's priceless. In every example and every little procedure, the benefits of treatment have the potential to be priceless.

If you can communicate this to your team, they will not only feel better about what they do, but they will have no problem collecting the dollars for the procedures provided.

Dentistry is only expensive if you don't see it as valuable and necessary for a good life. If you don't think dentistry is important, then you don't belong on my team, plain and simple.

Simple Vehicles and Clear Policies

In order to finance patients, everyone on the team needs to know what your financial policies are. You need to create clear policies so that everyone is on the same page. Every single person in your office should know how to create a financial contract and set it up.

At my practice, we use two outside financing companies: Lending Club and SimplePay. We lead with Lending Club, but if their credit is bad and they get denied, we move on to SimplePay. If they aren't approved for either, they'll have to wait until they can finance treatment.

There are special situations where we will do in-house financing for a patient. If the patient has a copay of under $500, we will allow them to make two or three payments, but only if it is a recurring charge on the credit or debit card. We do not mail statements every month hoping they will mail a check. Also, in orthodontics, we will allow them to spread payments over the course of treatment, but they must be auto recurring on a bank or credit card.

For normal procedures, the patient has three choices for financing:

- Pay in full
- Finance with an outside company
- Make payments if under $500 or doing orthodontics

That's it. Now I just need to teach my team how to use my two outside lenders, Lending Club and Simple Pay, and know how to set up an in-office payment plan on a recurring charge if the conditions are met.

There is no reason why everyone on your team can't be trained to do this.

Never Present Finances Over the Front Desk

You need a private area in which you can discuss finances with the patient. If you have a consult room, you need to use it for that. Presenting treatment over the front desk is a sure case killer. The patient and the presenter should be sitting down in a quiet environment where they can communicate and get the patient what they need to make it work for them.

What about presenting in the operatories with the patient in the chair? The only time this is acceptable is for same-day treatment, because you want to keep the patient in the chair. If you walk them to the front and they can see that door, they have a higher chance of wanting to reschedule and leave. If you are not doing the treatment the same day, go over all finances in the consult room.

What if you don't have a consult room? It's time to create one. What if you don't have extra space to make one? Then it's time to get rid of the doctor's office or clean it up so it can be used for consults.

You absolutely need a room!

Ballpark Fees

How would you feel if someone who was going to sell you something couldn't personally tell you what it would cost? I would think that possibly that person knows the product doesn't justify the price, and they are uncomfortable with it.

I am not saying that you need to get in a long financial discussion. However, there is no reason why you can't explain to the patient that fees are different depending on what insurance you have, but a ballpark estimate is around X dollars, and insurances might cover a portion of that. Explain that your treatment coordinator will give an actual breakdown and will provide financing options if needed. Tell the patient that you want to focus on what they need, and all of their financial questions will be answered shortly.

For Larger Treatments, Quote a Payment, Not a Price

At my practice everyone knows what we call *The Big 3*. The Big 3 are the monthly payments on an implant start to finish, an Invisalign case, and an eight-unit veneer case. We just went to Lending Club's website and found this.

EXTENDED PLANS

TERM	MONTHLY PAYMENT DUE	APR	PRACTICE FEE
60 months	$74 - $107	7.99% - 24.99%	$215.64 (5.99%)
48 months	$87 - $121	6.99% - 24.99%	$215.64 (5.99%)
36 months	$110 - $145	5.99% - 24.99%	$215.64 (5.99%)
24 months	$157 - $195	3.99% - 24.99%	$215.64 (5.99%)

The fee for an Invisalign case:

TERM	MONTHLY PAYMENT DUE	APR	PRACTICE FEE
60 months	$98 - $143	7.99% - 24.99%	$287.52 (5.99%)
48 months	$119 - $161	6.99% - 24.99%	$287.52 (5.99%)
36 months	$147 - $193	5.99% - 24.99%	$287.52 (5.99%)
24 months	$209 - $259	3.99% - 24.99%	$287.52 (5.99%)

The fee for an 8 unit veneer case:

TERM	MONTHLY PAYMENT DUE	APR	PRACTICE FEE
60 months	$163 - $238	7.99% - 24.99%	$399.20 (4.99%)
48 months	$193 - $268	6.99% - 24.99%	$399.20 (4.99%)
36 months	$244 - $322	5.99% - 24.99%	$399.20 (4.99%)
24 months	$348 - $432	3.99% - 24.99%	$399.20 (4.99%)

The actual payment terms will be determined by credit and length of financing. By using the lowest payment, and rounding it to an easy number, our *Big 3* then are $75, $100, and $170 a month for an implant, Invisalign case, or eight-unit veneer case, respectively.

Everyone on your team needs to know these. When a patient asks how much it would cost to do a smile makeover on their top teeth and you are planning on eight veneers, you can say, "It will depend on your insurance coverage ultimately, but most people finance them at around $170/month." Then shut up. That's all you need to say.

What if you said, "It's going to cost $7800." You would rarely if ever close that case. Most dentists I know couldn't come up with $7800 without financing.

Pick three large procedures that you want everyone to know the monthly cost on, and then quiz them on it from time to time. By using payments and being comfortable enough to quote a fee as the doctor, your treatment acceptance will go up immediately with these larger cases.

Get the Payment as Low as Possible

As shown on the charts from Lending Club, it makes no difference in fees when you extend payment from 24 months to 60 months. Why not quote the lowest number, which would be 60 months? All you need to do is find a monthly payment that works in the patient's budget, instead of hoping the patient has the full amount sitting in a checking account and is ready to part with it.

Summarize the Treatment and Don't Itemize

When our practice management systems print out treatment plans, they can be overwhelming. A tooth that needs a root canal will also need a build up and crown. Perio treatment is listed by quadrant and each quadrant has additional codes for irrigation or antibiotic placement. You will need to give the patient a copy of the treatment plan, but if your PMS allows, only print the summary numbers and not a price for each individual item.

Also, when your treatment coordinator is talking to the patient, they should summarize the treatment. Never list everything verbally like, "Tooth #2 needs a three-surface filling, #3 a build up and crown, #4 a root canal, buildup, and crown" etc. This means nothing to the patient. Summarize it, tell them what insurance will pay, and then tell them their total out of pocket as a monthly payment. You might say, "Here is a list of the recommended treatment. Your insurance will pay $920. We can get all of your treatment completed for around $120 a month." Then stop. You need to give the patient time to respond or make an objection. This is one of those situations in which the next person to talk loses.

The patient is often surprised that their insurance doesn't cover more. Sometimes they want to know more about the financing. Other times they will say they need to think about it. Either way, you need to let them respond. Which brings us to our next section on objections.

Objections

Nobody likes the dentist. It's very easy for patients to find other things to spend their money on. Many times they will say they need to discuss it with their spouse, think about it, or say they are really busy and need to get back to us. Usually these responses are just a polite way of saying no and getting out of there. The treatment coordinator needs to try to find out what their actual objection is so that they can address it. Objections usually are centered on four things: money, insurance, fear, or time/inconvenience.

Money

Sometimes patients just don't have the money, and that's OK. You will never overcome that objection when it's true. However, what they won't tell you is that they are going to the Bahamas next month, or buying a new car, or basically, that they would rather spend their money other places that are more fun and rewarding to them. If that is the case, the treatment coordinator should reinforce the idea that problems are only going to get worse and become more painful and expensive to fix down the road. They should offer financing again, but don't push too hard.

Insurance

When patients make comments about insurance, the TC should explain how dental insurance is very different from medical insurance. We often tell patients that medical is great for big things like surgeries, but really bad for small things like exams and labs. Dental insurance, however, is really great for the small things, but not good for the larger treatments. It is really only a discount plan, and while it is good that they pay something, it never covers nearly as much as we would prefer. You can then show the patient on their treatment plan where their insurance benefits run out because of the yearly maximum. Hopefully they will see that they have a lot of treatment remaining and relying on insurance benefits would take years and things would only get worse.

Fear

If the patient is fearful, the TC needs to empathize with those concerns. Offer sedation. The benefits are great, especially if you do oral conscious or IV. The patient can go to sleep and wake up when everything is completed. How great does that sound?

Time/Inconvenience

Again, empathize with them. People are busy. Remember that the time and inconvenience is only going to increase if they wait. This is another great opportunity to offer sedation, as they can get all of their treatment done in one visit most of the time.

The treatment coordinator needs to be a detective. If the patient is not disclosing much about what their true objection is, ask a good open ended question. An example would be, "Tell me how you are feeling about all of this right now?" or,

"If money was not an issue, would there be anything else keeping you from proceeding with treatment?" These are not hard sell techniques and the TC has to have enough social skills to know not to push too hard. A lot of times, the doctor really didn't convince the patient it was important to do the treatment. You can't blame the patient.

Putting Out the Fires

Putting out the fires is part of my practice's culture. Basically, we as a team all understand that caries or tooth decay is caused by acid in the patient's mouth. It comes from diet, but also very much from natural bacteria living in our mouths. Our saliva buffers that acid, but when we have a lot of decay, the environment of our mouths becomes constantly acidic, until we take care of all the tooth decay. When the environment is that acidic, all the good bacteria die because they cannot live in that environment, and the bad bacteria overpopulate. Then the snowball effect begins. The decay progresses more rapidly and spreads to all of the teeth. If we cannot get them back to baseline, the cavities will spread back to the teeth we have already fixed. We need to treat it as a disease, which it is.

That is the sole reason why we advocate for not waiting for insurance renewals, and not spreading out treatment too far. Everyone on your team should understand the etiology of caries.

There is one other thing that I often factor into my treatment planning. Ideal treatment is best, but we're not living in an ideal world. We're not treating 'the perfect patient.' We're treating real patients. They don't always prioritize dental health the way we think they ought to, and they don't always have the means to afford the treatment they need. If you put patients in the 'ideal treatment trap,' they may never get the work completed. So it's important to create treatment options that they're willing to accept, can afford, and that will effect a real, positive change in their oral health, even if you can't do it with the ideal or best treatment plan.

The treatment coordinator and financing is critical to getting out of tooth-by-tooth dentistry and moving towards comprehensive care. Spend time discussing your expectations with the people on your front end who will be presenting treatment. Get them the training they need to be effective. There are many resources available in our field for them to become better at leading the patients to say yes. If you do your part on the clinical end by conveying the need, a trained treatment coordinator should have no problem getting treatment acceptance in the consult room.

The TC should be able to change the treatment plans for the patient to make them more affordable if the patient wants. This is not belittling our treatment plan, but making it work within the patient's budget to get them happy and healthy again. The patient needs a root canal, build up, and crown to restore the tooth that brought them in. A lot of dentists would treat this tooth, but is that really the right thing for the patient? I think it is more important to look at the entire mouth. Let's say this patient has many other teeth in bad shape. I think the patient should know this, so that they can decide what to do comprehensively.

I like to tell the patient, that if by doing this root canal, they use all their available finances so that they cannot treat the other caries and gum disease, I would rather extract that tooth and "spread the love" across more teeth in their mouth.

You and I both know that if we just do one root canal, it doesn't take care of the etiology of the rampant decay. Nothing is more shaming to the profession than doing a full mouth extraction on a bunch of teeth that have had root canals and crowns because the decay was always rampant and the risk factors never discussed. The patient was in the chair, they spent the money on their teeth, and it failed, because their dentist did tooth-by-tooth dentistry instead of discussing comprehensive care and risk factors.

Or, think about socket preservation. We know it is best to preserve the bone after an extraction, but again, it is optional for the most part if finances are an issue and if the patient cannot afford to replace the tooth anyway. A broken tooth can be restored with a MODFL composite instead of a crown most of the time. A giant composite is better than a giant cavity on someone with rampant decay.

Don't let your patients down by not treating their entire mouth. It's easy to make a quick buck when the patient is in pain and will do the root canal that same day, but is it really the right thing when the patient has no idea what additional treatment is needed elsewhere in their mouth? I think not. Do the right thing.

I remember taking out nine lower teeth that all had root canals, but no crowns. They were fractured and broken; the endos were failing and unrestorable. This patient was someone that paid for nine root canals and buildups, to try to save her teeth. She spent the money, sat in the chair, and went through the dentistry, yet she still lost those teeth. If the dentist would have expressed the need for comprehensive care and risk factors, she may have been able to keep her teeth, as she obviously valued dentistry. She showed up. The dentist failed.

I don't care what you think; I honestly believe that caries control as a bunch of extractions and a partial is a better treatment plan than one root canal and crown while leaving the other diseased teeth unattended. Think about that. Don't fail your patients! Educate them and let them decide what is best for them. Don't ever go for the easy buck because it is sitting right in front of you; instead do what is right for the patient. Stop treating teeth and start treating mouths.

Homework

- Just write down this simple statement: "I resolve to stop treating individual teeth and begin treating entire mouths." Then live it.

- Talk to your team and create clear financial policies that everyone understands.

Find the dollar amount for your "Big 3", then start quizzing your team on it so they know these numbers by heart.

CHAPTER 16
THE TRUE TEST—SCHEDULING

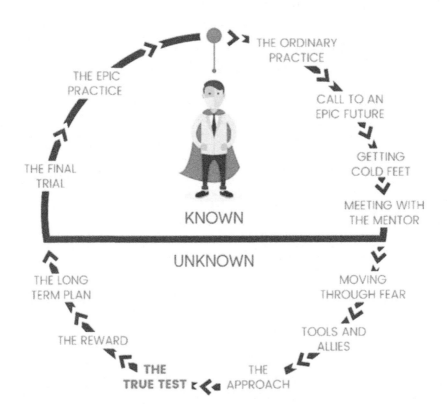

THE ORDINARY PRACTICE

THE EPIC PRACTICE

CALL TO AN EPIC FUTURE

GETTING COLD FEET

THE FINAL TRIAL

MEETING WITH THE MENTOR

KNOWN

UNKNOWN

THE LONG TERM PLAN

MOVING THROUGH FEAR

THE REWARD

TOOLS AND ALLIES

THE TRUE TEST

THE APPROACH

You've gotten the treasure, or at least an IOU for the treasure, but your heroic ordeal isn't over yet. Scheduling is a key part of productivity, efficiency, and ultimately great PX. Without an effective scheduling method, your practice will be in chaos, you'll work too hard, you'll fail to meet production goals, and you'll create the kind of experience that makes your staff unhappy and your patients abandon you for better offices. With a great schedule, on the other hand, you'll be relaxed and confident, your office will run-on time and with an air of calm, and your patients and staff will have an excellent experience every time they cross your threshold.

Out of all the systems in this book, scheduling may be the easiest to understand and the hardest to implement. It requires your front desk to have the verbal skills to schedule the patients in specific places that result in relaxed and high-producing days.

I can tell you from experience that nothing has changed my practice more than changing the way we schedule. At any given moment at my practice, there is one doctor, two hygienists, two assistants, two front desk people, and a treatment coordinator. Before we switched to block scheduling, we used to produce anywhere from $4000 to $7000 a day before write offs. When we started block scheduling, we immediately jumped to $12,000 to $15,000 a day. We've more than doubled it at a time when I really felt that we couldn't possibly squeeze any more production out of our existing hours. The great thing about block scheduling is that you produce more, and you don't work as hard. You can easily double your production just by changing the way you schedule, as long as your new patient, patient experience, treatment acceptance, and financing systems are working well.

Because we block schedule, I can often produce in three days what most people do in five or six. At the time of this writing, we just finished our sixth month of the year, June, and I have produced over $650,000 in my doctor chairs on 22 clinical hours a week. That gives me more time off and allows me to pay my staff better, as well as afford the technologies that I want my practice to have.

It's important to realize that high numbers are really not about money, they are about freedom. If the numbers are good, we have the freedom to live our lives in a way that we desire and enjoy. Also, good numbers show that your practice is running efficiently, and if you are selling ethically, you are helping a lot more people in less time. Everyone wins!

Think of how much your life would change if you produced more in less time. You could easily cut down on your days and take more weeks of vacation. You could have more time to work on your practice instead of in it. You could spend more time with your family or hobbies that you love. You could take the time to volunteer or go on dental mission trips to help people in other countries. Being more productive while we are at work opens a whole new realm of possibility!

Scheduling Makes the Practice

Traditional or provider time scheduling creates days that are a patchwork of many small appointments. I remember one day in which I did 34 direct composites on around twenty different patients. I can tell you that we ran like hell that day, and when I got home I was completely burnt out. To make matters worse, a day full of composites isn't a very big day. So essentially, traditional or provider scheduling makes you work really hard, and for little production.

Remember that a great practice operates with very little stress. Having a lot of small unproductive appointments in your schedule as you bounce from room to room is stressful. Sure it's very easy to train the staff on how to schedule in this manner, but I assure you this type of scheduling does not serve you or your team.

The Power of the Block

Scheduling in blocks is a much more difficult type of schedule to implement, mostly because there isn't as much flexibility in where you can place patient appointments. It's not as easy as just putting any appointment anywhere it fits.

There are two important principles to realize in this model:

1. We strategically block out portions of our schedule. These blocks cannot be negotiated; they are fundamental to our schedule running smoothly and productively.

2. We give the patient options for appointments that fit with our schedule, not the other way around.

Block-outs

Go in your schedule, and start placing three types of block-outs.

*   **Major Blocks** – These are the high production blocks; they are for crowns, root canals, implants, full mouth extractions, multiple incisal composites, and anything else that is high production. This is not the place for fillings.

*   **Minor Blocks** – These are for the smaller things that are less productive, like fillings.

*   **Other blocks** – These are very specific blocks. We use them for ortho adjustments and molar root canals. Hygiene has blocks for SRP's, recall, and new patients. You can use whatever blocks you want. Start with something and start finding what works in your practice. The reason that molar root canals are a separate block for me is that I need a little more time for a molar root canal than what I have in one of my major blocks.

Weekly Variations

My schedule has four variations of the blocks for each week of the month, so that if a patient needs a specific time, you can keep moving forward and hopefully one of the weekly variations will have the proper block in the proper time. Notice that the later, more high demand, hours for hygiene are blocked as well.

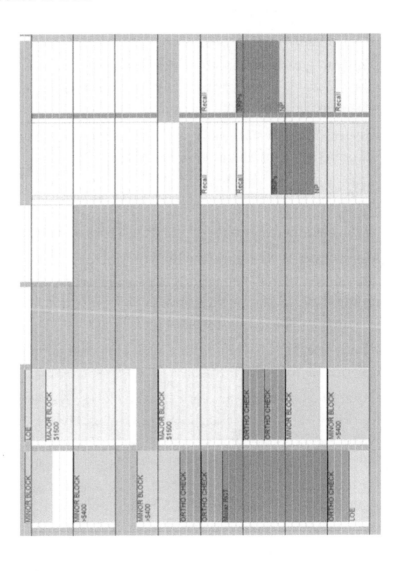

Major PM

LOE

MINOR BLOCK
>$400

MINOR BLOCK
>$400

MAJOR BLOCK
$1500

ORTHO CHECK

ORTHO CHECK

MINOR BLOCK
>$400

ORTHO CHECK

LOE

Recall

TNP

Recall

ORTHO CHECK

MAJOR BLOCK
$1500

ORTHO CHECK

MINOR BLOCK
>$400

TNP

Recall

Billing

TNP

MAJOR BLOCK $1500

LOE

MINOR BLOCK >$400

LOE

MINOR BLOCK >$400

MINOR BLOCK >$400

ORTHO CHECK

ORTHO CHECK

MAJOR BLOCK $1500

MINOR BLOCK >$200

MAJOR BLOCK $1500

MINOR BLOCK >$400

MINOR BLOCK >$200

ORTHO CHECK

NP

EXAMS

Recall

Recall

Recall

STOP

Recall

Recall

Recall
NO X-RAYS

MINOR BLOCK >$400

LOE

MINOR BLOCK >$400

MINOR BLOCK SINGLE FILLING

LOE

MINOR BLOCK >$400

ORTHO CHECK

MAJOR BLOCK $1500

MINOR BLOCK >$400

ORTHO CHECK

ORTHO CHECK

MAJOR BLOCK $1500

MAJOR BLOCK $1500

ORTHO CHECK

Recall

Recall

Recall

NP

Recall

Recall

NP

NP

Recall

Schedules are Made to be Adjusted

Your new schedule is a work in progress. You can always alter and change it. Where my blocks are now was the result of trial and error, and it is what works for my office. You need to discover your own rhythm, but you need to start somewhere, so get out that schedule and start blocking.

For example, I ran some reports and found that I do a molar RCT about 1.5 times a week on average. We set up our Molar RCT blocks to follow that. If I find that I am booking out really far in the future for that procedure, I will need to add more.

I have two to three major blocks each day. That is a result of us trying to have five major blocks a day and not filling those. It has to work with what you diagnose and your patient flow.

The most important principle is that you start with a template, and then modify and readjust course as time goes on. Ready, Fire, Aim!

Filling Your Major Blocks

Obviously, if you can't fill your major blocks, you likely have another problem—either lack of treatment acceptance or lack of diagnosis. If those are in check though, you will have no problem filling the major blocks.

The minor blocks will be the easiest to fill. The majority of what you diagnose will be fillings. Let's face it, that's the reality. What is going to happen is that your minor blocks will fill up very far out; I am talking to the point of three or four months sometimes. All the while you will have massive amounts of open time in your major blocks. As you can imagine, some patients will freak out about waiting three months to get their fillings. I always like to tell the patient when they need fillings, "These aren't urgent to the point that we need to fix them this week, but make sure you get them done before your next cleaning." By telling them this, they understand that little to no harm is done by waiting awhile to get back in for their fillings. We also have an ASAP list of patients to call when we have cancellations so that they can get in earlier if a space opens up.

Don't let the major blocks being open scare you. They will fill. Someone will call the day before to schedule the crown. They almost always do, at least in my experience. If the idea of leaving all that time open in your days scares you, then maybe choose only half of the day to schedule in this manner. Maybe start with just one day per week. See what happens. After trying it, I know you will be hooked.

Blocking time for high production procedures will immediately give your daily production a boost. The problem with not blocking things, is that the days will fill up with a lot of little non-productive appointments first, and you will be forced to schedule far out for your crowns and major things. That is backwards and not the way we want to do it. Just give it a try.

If you find that after you block-schedule your day you're sitting around a lot, reduce the length of your major blocks or add some more minor blocks. If you find yourself working too hard, make your blocks longer or more spaced out. Find what works for you and your practice. It's an evolution. Great scheduling looks different for every dentist, because a great schedule is tailored to your vision for the practice and your preference for each day.

Blocking for Hygiene

Hygiene needs to have portions of their days blocked out for new patients and perio treatments. You need to designate this time; otherwise recall patients will fill the schedule and you won't have anywhere to put new patients or schedule someone for quads of scaling. Scaling and root planing is the most productive hygiene procedure there is. Don't let your existing patients' recall appointments keep your hygienists from being able to schedule perio treatment or see new patients.

Change is Hard

When you first implement this, your front desk is bound to be upset. You need to be persistent and watch how your schedules fill so that you can monitor the blocks and make sure that your schedulers are respecting them.

We got really lax about respecting the blocks for a while. Our days were feeling very busy and less productive. What happened was that one person would violate a block by placing something that didn't belong in it, which gave the next person a reason to not obey that particular block because it was already screwed up. We had to go back to the basics and make sure that all blocks were obeyed at all times.

Block scheduling is like dominos if you disobey. Catch these mistakes early so that you can reschedule patients or move blocks around. And get your front office staff the training and verbal skills they need to make this happen. Try a consultant that is familiar with this type of scheduling.

I said earlier that this is easy to understand but harder to implement, but have faith. If you are persistent about it, it will change, and then it will be smooth sailing.

Homework

Find the next day that is open on your schedule and place a few blocks in it. Then, have a team meeting discussing how to block schedule and what can go where. Get clear on what you want your schedule to look like.

CHAPTER 17

THE TRUE TEST—PX DURING TREATMENT

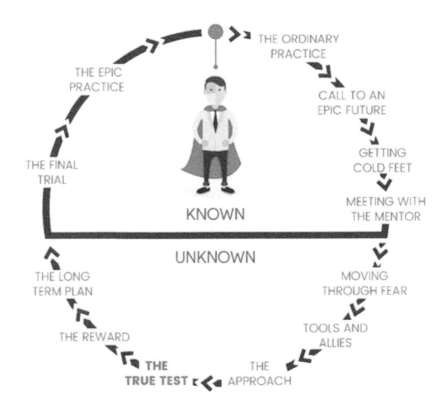

THE ORDINARY PRACTICE

THE EPIC PRACTICE

CALL TO AN EPIC FUTURE

THE FINAL TRIAL

GETTING COLD FEET

MEETING WITH THE MENTOR

KNOWN

UNKNOWN

THE LONG TERM PLAN

MOVING THROUGH FEAR

THE REWARD

TOOLS AND ALLIES

THE TRUE TEST

THE APPROACH

It's a rare patient who needs one thing, once in their life, and never needs anything again. It's an even rarer patient who doesn't have friends and family who need treatment. Even at the moment where you're placing an implant or working on a root canal, your patient's experience matters. A Heroic Dentist combines clinical excellence with a human touch so that after a procedure the patient can get up and say, "Gee, Doc, that wasn't as bad as I was expecting!"

Once you have treatment acceptance, financing, and scheduling under control, it's time to execute the treatment plan. Patients want you to handle treatment efficiently, because no one wants to spend longer in the chair than they have to.

When you have better systems for case acceptance, you can increase production by having more patients say yes. You can start keeping more cases in-house instead of referring them out, and you can schedule your blocks efficiently so you're not running around constantly switching gears all day.

The Supergeneralist—A Dental Hero

This is the idea of the supergeneralist. There are so many CE and online resources for you to expand your skill set. What's even better is that if you are only doing restorative procedures, chances are you have a lot of openings in your daily schedule.

People always ask me how my schedule stays booked out so far. The answer is I am supergeneralist. I still refer to specialists, but I do about 85% of molar endos; place most implants; do ortho on adults, adolescents, and children; administer botox; do all surgical extractions minus third molars; and do bone grafting.

As a general dentist, we are licensed to perform practically any specialty procedure under the sun. Think of our friends in the medical field. You won't find your primary care physician taking courses so that she can perform heart surgery or Brazilian butt lifts.

Some people argue that the specialist can do it better. I would say that's partially true. They do the same thing all day long. But the fact of the matter is that patients don't want to go to the specialist. They like and trust you and would rather you do it even if they know someone could do it better. Know how to kill a case? Tell the patient you need them to get some teeth extracted before you do any of the other work and send them to the specialist.

They aren't going unless it hurts, trust me!

One of the coolest things for me is when I prep a crown, scan it with CEREC, and have my assistant making the crown while I do the endo. The whole appointment takes around two hours. Let's imagine this patient has had an endo before, where her GP referred her to the endo, and then she returned to her GP, had a temp crown, and then returned to the GP again to get it cemented. How different is the experience of having it all done at one place in around two hours? Can you say "WOW!"

If you are a general dentist and all you do is restorative work, are you really even a general dentist? No, because you *generally* only do restorative. You're kind of like a triage dentist, who happens to know how to restore teeth.

Dentists need to take CE.

In Illinois we only have to take 36 CE hours every three years. That's a joke. The greatest investment you can ever make, more than anything you do in real estate or the stock market, is to invest in your skill set and do it early. If you are right out of school, forego buying the fancy car and use the money saved to drop $20k on CE.

Get into the Growth Zone

I am not advocating being cavalier with your patient treatment; I am just saying to expand your horizons on what you offer to people. If you think about it, no matter how much training you receive, you are never really 100% proficient when you try a new procedure. Do you think you were qualified to perform fillings on patients in dental school when you first tried? Not really. We practiced on model teeth quite a bit, but when we got to the mouth, it was a different story.

In dental school though, we had instructors to push us past our limits to be better. I remember one of my first amalgams I placed was on #15 on a person with a small mouth that really couldn't open very far. I told my instructor I couldn't see while I was drilling. He told me that, "sometimes you can't see when you are drilling; figure it out!" I remember how worn out I was after cutting my prep for two hours.

We need to get outside of our comfort zone in order to grow. Now that we are out of dental school, the only person that is going to push us there is ourselves. As Master Shifu in *Kung Fu Panda 3* said, "If you only do what you can do, you'll never be better than what you are."

This is what most "General Dentists" do. They stick with what they know, for the fear of getting uncomfortable. Essentially, they are complacent or scared.

Take your patient care and income to new heights. Constantly push the envelope while knowing better than to get into the danger zone. Sure, you're going to do some things during your growth that you hope no one else will see, but the fact of the matter is that you grow from learning from your mistakes. The worst thing you can do in your dental career is stay stagnant. As Tony Robbins says, "If you aren't growing, you're dying."

Twenty years of the same experience is not equal to twenty

years of growth experience. Don't doubt yourself or let fear get the best of you. You can do this! You are a Hero, after all!

Use Your Team to the Fullest Extent

Your dental practice is a business, and you need to be spending most of your time doing what brings in money. No one in the office will produce as much as the doctor. Even all of your super-hygienists combined will produce only a third to half of what you as one doctor will. The doctor needs to be busy producing.

You need to really look at the dental practice laws in your state, and see what your auxiliaries and hygienists are licensed to do, then train them on how to do all those things the way you would do them.

Let's use an example of two doctors: Dr. Great and Dr. Efficient. Dr. Great is really good at his crowns. He is an occlusion expert, and his temporaries are perfect, almost as good as the final crowns. His contacts are perfect and his margins as well. He is great at hitting all of his blocks; he never misses.

Dr. Great seats his crown patient at 8AM. He anesthetizes and waits ten minutes. He then spends 40 minutes refining his crown and getting everything just the way he wants. He takes an impression, then makes the temporary. It is now 9AM. He cements his temporary and gets it all dialed in, post ops his patient, and leaves for his next appointment at 9:20AM. His visit only took an hour and twenty minutes.

He then sees the patient for the seat appointment. He anesthetizes, removes his temp, and starts making adjustments; he cleans the crown and disinfects the tooth; he cements it and cleans all the cement off. He then checks the bite another time. Everything is perfect as he expected. This visit took about 40 minutes, bringing the total time he spent with the patient to two hours.

Now let's look at Dr. Efficient. His RDH seats and anesthetizes the patients at 7:50AM. Dr. Efficient walks in at 8AM and starts prepping; he is done with his prep at 8:15; he takes the impression and leaves the room, letting the assistant hold it in the mouth. He is in the next room working on his next patient at 8:25. His assistant then makes the temporary, adjusts it, and cements it. They are done at 9:00 AM. Dr. Efficient finishes his other patient and pops in to say goodbye and thank the patient. He spent only about 15-20 minutes in the room today.

The patient arrives for their crown seat; the RDH anesthetizes; the assistant removes the temporary, adjusts the new crown, cleans it out, disinfects the prep, isolates, and pages the doctor. The doctor comes in, squirts the cement in the crown, and pushes it down on the tooth and then leaves back to his other patient. After the assistant cleans up the cement, takes a post-cementation X-ray, and gives the patient the post op instructions, the doctor returns to check the occlusion and thanks the patient. He spent less than five minutes on this appointment. This brings his total time in the room for the crown to 25 minutes vs. Dr. Great who spent two hours.

Who got a better result? They were equal. If you don't believe that, you need to really think about how easy some things we do in dentistry are. If you think you need four years of dental school to make a great temporary, adjust the crown, get it ready to cement, and clean the cement off, you are out of your mind. These skills can be taught to your assistants and if you check their results and train them, you can get them to do it just as good as you.

Some of us don't like to run from room to room, and that's fine. I have days where I am a little slow, but I am still not making temps and adjusting crowns. I am doing other things like working on my practice. In my practice we have CEREC, and I delegate all the crown fabrication to my assistants. I am already out of the room working on another patient.

You need to take the time to train your clinical staff. Upfront it is a little more work, but the time saving and production increase it allows is worth it. I didn't mention that Dr. Great is fee for service and Dr. Efficient takes a PPO with a 30% write off. Dr. Great got paid $1200 for his crown. Dr. Efficient did three additional crowns in the time that Dr. Great did one, and got paid $3,360 for them. I am not advocating for PPO's, but using this example you can see how even if Dr. Efficient was on a PPO that had a 50% reduction, he still produced more money by $1200. In case you were wondering, my practice at the present time is contracted with three PPO's. We continue to drop them each time we reach a capacity point and hope to drop another very soon. Our write off is around 20%.

Another thing I left out is that Dr. Great probably writes his own clinical notes and lab slips. Assistants can do this as well. Hygienists can write all of your exam notes. At the end of the day you can check them, which only takes a few minutes. If you are going to get uber-efficient with your production, you are not going to want to waste your time doing paperwork.

All it takes is training, checking, and coaching them to write everything the exact same way as you would.

One more thing about training your clinical staff to their full extent: they will love their job so much more when they are actually contributing something more than suctioning. Every assistant I have ever trained has told me that. I promise if I ever lost an assistant to another practice for some reason, the doctor that acquired her would be the luckiest dentist in the world. My assistants are absolutely amazing, but we never started that way with any of them.

Same Day Dentistry

When is the best time to do dental work for a patient that is in our office? NOW! It is never more convenient for the patient than the day they are already there for recall or their new patient exam. They are off work, they have a sitter, their motivation is high, and they almost always have the time to stick around a little longer to get something done. They are already in the chair! Just offer it and get it done!

You can easily add $1500 or more in same day dentistry every day. One day we added almost $9,000 with an Invisalign start and a few crowns.

Also, a good way to keep your future schedule clear of single fillings and small non-productive stuff, is to do it same day. If I ever plan a single restoration, I try to get it done right there. The patient wins by saving them time and another trip, and I win because I just collected more money than I had scheduled that day.

Organizing Your Rooms for Efficiency

If you want to be able to pound out some same-day things in between your patients, you need to work efficiently. That means your RDH is getting the patient numb while your assistant is setting up the procedure.

I love that my team can get an endo set up in less than five minutes using the cart. You never know what is going to show up at the dental office each day. Be ready to treat the patient right there and they will be very much appreciative that you were able to make it happen for them.

Now that we have gotten our patient through our machine and produced the dentistry, all that is left is to collect the money and send the patient back through the system again.

Homework

List three ways you can use your team and your time better. Then come up with a next actionable step for each of these changes.

CHAPTER 18
THE TRUE TEST—COLLECTING YOUR PAY

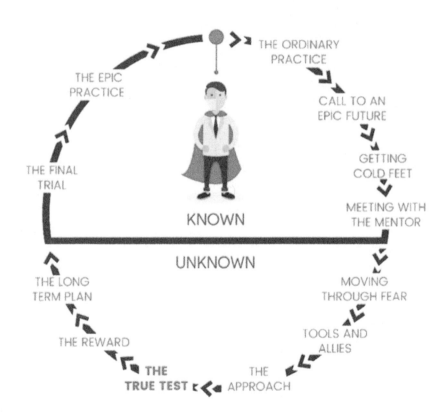

THE ORDINARY PRACTICE

THE EPIC PRACTICE

CALL TO AN EPIC FUTURE

THE FINAL TRIAL

GETTING COLD FEET

KNOWN

MEETING WITH THE MENTOR

UNKNOWN

THE LONG TERM PLAN

MOVING THROUGH FEAR

THE REWARD

TOOLS AND ALLIES

THE TRUE TEST

THE APPROACH

Every single part of this book up to this point means nothing if you cannot collect the dollars that you produce on. A solid practice should be collecting at a level of at least 98%. I have heard of practices from talking to consultants that are collecting at levels that would make the worst dentist cringe. I have heard of practices that bill everyone after the claim closes and don't collect a penny until months later.

If you don't collect on the dollars you produce, you are essentially providing charity work. We all know that the last person to be paid will always be the dentist. I can even say that recently I was sent a final notice before collection action for a $260 medical bill from my primary care physician. It wasn't that I couldn't afford it, but rather that when I received the statement each month, it often got thrown in a pile for things to do later when I had time. Unfortunately, that time never came until I received the collections letter. The balance was over six months old.

I haven't had a late payment to a credit card or my mortgage in probably a decade. Why is it so easy for me to pay them but I can't pay my doctor? I know I am not alone. It is because doctors and dentists offices are generally soft when it comes to collections.

I know that if my mortgage is 15 days late, they will be calling me. I know that if I am late on my credit card they will be calling, and it could very well affect my credit score in a negative way.

So if I, as someone who works in health care, can't pay my doctor on time, how I can expect my patients to pay my office if I am not collecting on the spot? The fact of the matter is I can't. Dental offices can't afford to bill as ineffectively as medical offices do. We need to conquer the problem of patient balances.

Patient balances come from three avenues:

- Incorrect insurance estimates
- Insurance denials
- Our supporting staff not collecting

I am assuming that every office collects on the day of service. There are a few unicorns that collect before the appointment is even scheduled, and one day I hope to be one of those, but for now we collect the day of. Obviously, this is problematic, as patients will fail if they cannot come up with the copay, but for the majority of my patient base, this is not a problem.

If you are really good, have high demand, or offer a discount for prepaying, you can collect before the appointment is scheduled; but for the majority of us dentists, we fear if we make that our policy, our patients will go down the street where they can pay the day of or even worse, be billed for services. While some patients may cancel because they cannot come up with the copay, you should make your policies work for the majority of the patients and forget about the outliers.

Dealing with Incorrect Insurance Estimates

Incorrect insurance estimates drive patients nuts. They feel like they've been cheated. They were told one number, budgeted for it, and now you're telling them a different number. The incorrect estimates fall into one of two categories: either we made a mistake or the insurance company made a mistake.

We Made a Mistake

I already explained the importance of getting accurate insurance breakdowns and asking for all special clauses. We all know as dentists that it should be the patient's problem to understand all the special ins and outs of their insurance because after all, it is their insurance! The problem is that our patients do not feel the same. They don't understand insurance and for all they know, we have software that can run every possible scenario and tell them exactly what their copay will be.

If your team makes a mistake and doesn't ask for a clause, or a waiting period, or a posterior composite downgrade, and the patient is left with the balance, just honor the treatment plan that was presented, write off the rest, and make a note in the patient's chart so that you don't make the same mistake twice. Life is too short to try and collect these balances and it will never be worth the bad reviews or things those patients will say to their friends about you.

I mean it, *never*!

The Insurance Company Made a Mistake

Situations where the insurance company makes the mistake aren't much different than the ones where we make the mistake. The patient will always blame us. It only matters what the patient thinks in a world where someone can literally cost you thousands of dollars by writing a negative review about you.

Sometimes the insurance will tell you someone is active, only to retro-date back to the beginning of the month after the claim is sent, saying they actually were not. The insurance company can tell you that the patient doesn't have any special clauses, or that implants are covered, when in reality they aren't. Again, just honor the signed treatment plan you presented.

Once I met someone at a wedding. When a stranger finds out you are a dentist, they immediately want to ask you a dental question. Always leading with, "I know you probably don't want to talk about work stuff, but I got this thing…" You know how it goes. Anyway, the person had a crown break after a year and a half. Her dentist wouldn't replace it for her and her insurance had a five year replacement frequency. She was ticked because her dentist didn't warrant his services. She asked me if I warrant my crowns and if so, how long? I told her my warranty is as long as the patient thinks it is. That's the honest truth. If it has been two years and the patient is a bruxer for whom I have recommended some night protection and she declined it, I will tell her she broke it because she clenches and doesn't protect her teeth at night. I will then ask her, "What do you think is fair?" If she thinks I should replace for free, then that's what I am doing. I know a lot people may freak out about that, but my practice is doing well and has a fantastic reputation. That's worth more than refusing to do some free work for people now and then.

Know that I am not talking about large dollar amounts here. By large dollar amounts, I mean more than $1500, which is an average annual maximum in my area. That's the most I can really write off if the insurance doesn't pay. $1500 is really only like a crown and a filling. I can do that in thirty minutes, no big deal. How much time would you spend stressing over a negative review or someone coming into your waiting room screaming and yelling? Thirty minutes is getting off cheap.

If you really must collect on these, send a statement and see what the patient does. If they pay, great! If they call to complain, just write it off and be the good guy!

Small Differences in Estimates

Often there are small discrepancies in estimates that are under $100. For those we have a "small balance policy". What we do is have the patient sign a form saying that if the insurance payment is less than expected and less than $100, we will send a statement and if they do not pay, they give us authorization to charge the last card they used at our practice for that amount.

To do this you need a merchant service provider that can do this sort of thing. We are not storing their credit card numbers. The merchant services provider does that, and we just tell them what to charge. When the balance comes in, we send a statement with an orange piece of paper that says that if we do not hear from them in thirty days, we will charge their last credit card used at our office for their convenience. We also tell them that if they would like to use another form of payment, please contact us before the end of the month. We try to portray it as for their convenience and not ours. Make sure you use some neon paper for this.

We have been using this system for almost three years and have rarely gotten any pushback from patients about it. When I think about it, I wish my medical doctor would just charge my credit card. I love automatic bill pay and hate opening statements; that's why they sit in piles until I receive final notices!

Statements Cost More Than You Think

The problem with relying on statements to motivate the patient to pay is that they are pretty much ineffective for a lot of people until the final notice comes. That is usually after we send three to four statements and haven't heard from the patient.

If you think of the time it takes to audit the chart before sending a statement, the time to stuff the envelope, address it, and place a stamp on it, it could cost you $10-$20 in labor, and you may have to do the same thing next month. It is in our best interests to minimize the number of statements we send out.

Also, if the claim takes a while to close, and the patient has a small balance, they will be irritated that you are sending them a statement for something that they paid for already three or four months ago. They will feel like they need to check their records before they pay you as they already thought they were paid up. They will likely procrastinate doing this until they receive the final notice.

Insurance Denials

The second source of patient balances comes from the insurance denying payment on treatment because their "clinical consultant" has deemed it unnecessary and not approved for coverage. These are the most frustrating, because when you are ethically diagnosing and providing treatment, it really isn't the patient or the practitioner's fault. It's the patient's insurance company.

We handle these like a mistake in insurance breakdown. We honor the signed treatment plan and write off the difference as a courtesy for the patient. It's just my philosophy of practice. It's not worth the headache. We will try to appeal, but if our attempts fail, we will write it off.

Our Supporting Staff Did Not Collect

These are the most preventable patient balances. Basically, the patient said they couldn't pay today, and then we performed the work anyway. We used to check out restorative patients and collect payment after the procedure was complete. Eventually, we figured out that we need to collect before we do the treatment. When a patient checks in for anything other than routine preventative, we collect before they are called back to the operatory.

If they cannot pay, they go into the consult room to make arrangements. If they still cannot pay, we decide based on what the insurance will pay if it is more advantageous for us to accept the insurance money and hope that the patient will pay us later, or to reschedule the patient.

We usually base this decision on what else is going on in our schedule at that very moment. If we have other things to do, we will reappoint. If we have nothing else in the schedule, we will usually do the procedure if the insurance is paying for most of the treatment. If the patient never pays their part and we only collect the insurance money, it was still better than the zero dollars that we would have received if we reappointed them and didn't have anything else to do but sit on DentalTown for the next hour.

Get Credit for Your Write Offs

A lot of times when there is an insurance denial or frequency limitation that leaves the patient with a balance, the patient knows about it because they received their EOB. Even though you wrote the balance off, the patient may avoid you because they think they owe you money. Anytime you are going to forgive what the patient should rightfully owe you, you should call them to let them know that you wrote it off as a courtesy to them. It's always a great call for the patient to receive and will make sure that they appreciate your generosity instead of avoiding you.

Aging Insurance Claims

A single person in your office needs to be in charge of keeping up with unpaid insurance claims. If you have multiple people working on it, no one will. One person needs to be in charge of submitting the additional information the insurance requests, getting narratives written, and corresponding with the insurance on unpaid claims.

It is important for you, as the owner, to have a scheduled time every month in which you will look at the balances over 45-60 days. If you continue to audit and check the accounts receivable and aging insurance, your employee in charge of it will be held accountable to get those things taken care of.

Make sure you are taking intraoral photos, have the necessary radiographs, and supporting documentation in your notes so that your "insurance coordinator" will have what he/she needs to follow up on these claims.

Homework

Create some clear collection policies as a team. Get these in writing and make sure everyone understands them.

CHAPTER 19
THE REWARD AND THE LONG TERM PLAN

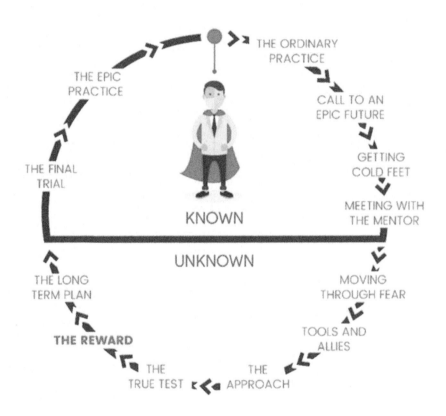

THE ORDINARY PRACTICE

THE EPIC PRACTICE

CALL TO AN EPIC FUTURE

GETTING COLD FEET

THE FINAL TRIAL

MEETING WITH THE MENTOR

KNOWN

UNKNOWN

THE LONG TERM PLAN

MOVING THROUGH FEAR

THE REWARD

TOOLS AND ALLIES

THE TRUE TEST

THE APPROACH

You've become a Dental Office hero who can provide excellent patient experience at each stage of the journey. Even your collections department provides a great experience, by minimizing the hassle for your patients, writing off discrepancies between the treatment plan and the final bill, and generally making your patients feel appreciated and valued. So where's your reward?

Because you treat your patients well, they return again and again and are more likely to accept treatment. They recommend your practice to family, friends, and that guy in line at the grocery store. You've created a corps of brand ambassadors, and you did it while focusing on the most interesting and entertaining parts of your practice. Work-life balance is around the corner, and you can enjoy the rewards of a shorter work week, better cash flow, and less stress. Congratulations, Hero.

THE LONG TERM PLAN

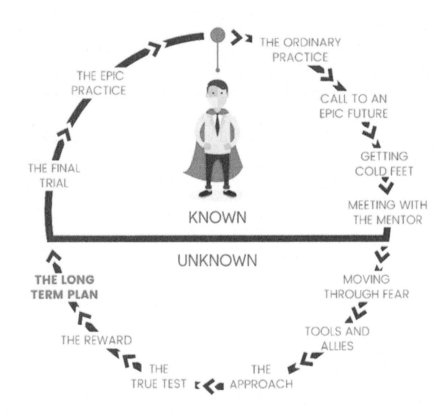

THE ORDINARY PRACTICE

THE EPIC PRACTICE

CALL TO AN EPIC FUTURE

GETTING COLD FEET

THE FINAL TRIAL

MEETING WITH THE MENTOR

KNOWN

UNKNOWN

THE LONG TERM PLAN

MOVING THROUGH FEAR

THE REWARD

TOOLS AND ALLIES

THE TRUE TEST

THE APPROACH

Adventures change a hero. You're no longer the callow youth who thought that marketing was about newspaper ads, that the only thing that matters is clinical skill, and that the schedule would take care of itself. You're a dental hero now. You can return home and enjoy the fruits of your labor as your systems keep the practice humming along. And, because your systems are in place, your patients will journey through your practice, over and over, for years to come.

If you can decrease your active patient attrition rate, your practice will continue to grow until you reach a capacity point, in which you can either increase the capacity or the value as discussed before. Making sure that patients stay active in your system is critical for this.

I can tell you from my experience that when you see a hundred new patients a month, you can easily lose sight of how many active patients you are losing. We did this for a long time until a consultant had me look at the number. I had never really paid any attention to it before.

While we were seeing around a hundred new patients a month, we were losing roughly 60-70 active patients each month. I honestly have no idea where they went. They may have gone to another office or just stopped going to the dentist altogether.

The problem with not paying attention to these numbers is that you never really realize that you may have a capacity issue. When we were seeing that many new patients, we didn't realize that if we could reappoint more of them and keep them in our system, we could have very well expanded much earlier. The whole idea is to grow your practice, and it's hard to do solely by having high new patient numbers.

The Doctor's Role

Explain at the end of each appointment what you would like the patient to schedule for next. For example, if a patient is finishing all of their restorative treatment and is to go back into the recare system, I will say to them, "Ok, Mrs. Jones, we are done with all of your recommended treatment. I want to see you back in August for your hygiene maintenance so we can check everything and make sure that we can address any new issues that may develop early, while they are small." It means more when the doctor is asking for it.

The Hygienist's Role

After each hygiene visit, the hygienist should explain to the patient when they are expected to come back for recall, what will be done at that visit, and why. By explaining what will be done at the next visit, we are creating value for the patient to return. The hygienist might say, "Ok, Mrs. Jones, we will see you back in August for your next hygiene visit. At that appointment, we will be taking X-rays to check for cavities between your teeth, perform your yearly oral cancer screening, and checking the health of your gum tissue." The hygienist should also be the one scheduling the appointment while they are waiting for the doctor or at the end of the visit, if they are not waiting. This establishes the personal relationship between the hygienist and the patient and makes it much more difficult for the patient to cancel or no show the appointment.

The Dental Assistants' Role

After seeing a patient in a doctor chair, the dental assistant should make sure the patient is scheduled for their recare appointment. No patient should ever leave without their next appointment scheduled.

When we graft an extraction site because we couldn't immediately place the implant, we schedule a post-op around three months out, to survey the bone for implant placement. We need to schedule that appointment while the patient is there. If we let them leave and tell them to call us when they are ready for the implant in four months, chances are life will happen and they will not.

The Front Office's Role

The front desk is responsible for making sure that all family members for anyone on our schedule have an appointment. This should be part of their daily duties and notes should be made on the schedule and routers for them to ask to schedule the family members without appointments.

Keeping Patients Active is a Team Sport

The best way to keep a patient from leaving your system is to not give them a reason to leave in the first place. Essentially, this is what this entire book has been about—having the systems in place so that your practice functions well, all while providing exceptional value to your patients.

Everyone should be responsible for working the reactivation list. If you check the list each month and make it a priority that all downtime will be spent following up on unscheduled treatment, as well as people who have become inactive, it will then be a priority for your team.

If you have a great practice culture in which everyone works together to better and grow the practice, it will be important to them as long as they understand why it is important. That's why looking at certain numbers and key performance indicators each month at your meeting is critical to practice growth.

What you measure will always improve, and what you audit will always get done. Never forget that if you don't care about things like reappointment and reactivation, your team won't either.

Homework

Find your active patient and attrition rates. Make a commitment as a team to improve upon these and review them at each meeting.

CHAPTER 20
THE FINAL TRIAL AND THE EPIC PRACTICE

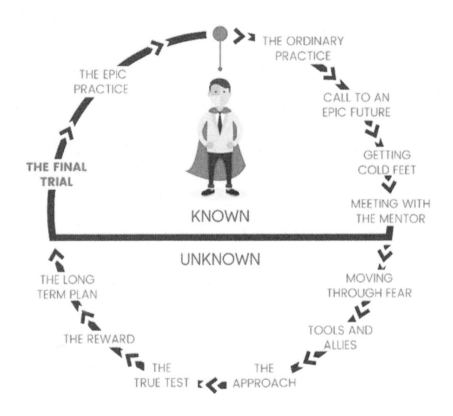

In the traditional hero's journey the hero faces one last, possibly fatal, foe as he returns home. He triumphs, because he has changed. What is your final foe?

You may think your work is done. You've done your homework. You've put great systems in place. Your practice should be perfect now, right?

Wrong. Remember when I talked about *Ready, Fire, Aim*? Your systems may be good and production might be soaring, but there's always room for improvement. Part of being a Hero to your practice is embracing a culture of continuous improvement. Keep looking around your office for sights, smells, sounds, and feelings that could be made more pleasing for your patients. Check the script of your drama to ensure it stays fresh and interesting. Look at your numbers, share them with the staff, and brainstorm ways to make your schedule even more productive. Commit yourself to a lifetime of improvement, and you'll keep your practice fresh, challenging, and fun.

THE EPIC PRACTICE

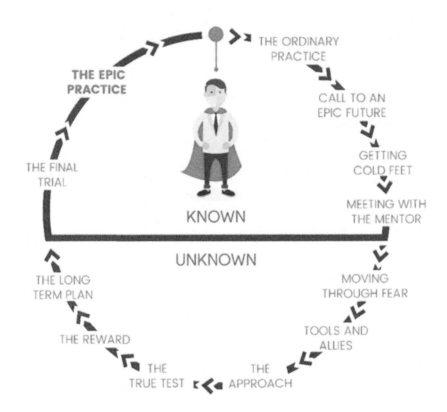

At last, the hero has returned home. He's completed the quest. He has time to tilt the work-life balance away from work and towards his home life. He can rest for a while, or he can use his new skills to transform his world. You have an epic practice. What will you do now that you've completed your journey?

Private practice dentistry is not dead. There has never been a better time for you to differentiate yourself from corporate as well as the other private practicing dentists that provide such a poor value to their patients.

As the title of this book said, your practice is ready for a hero.

A great dental machine does not get built overnight. There are so many elements to a great practice that when thought of properly and implemented, combine to produce an end result that is both awesome and extremely profitable.

Once the practice is extremely profitable, you as the owner will gain the freedom to live your life to its fullest extent possible by giving the people and things most important to you the time they deserve.

You are the driver of your own destiny. You are the owner. You are the hero. Everything at your practice will be a product of you and how much work you put into it. Your results will be based entirely on your thought process, organization of goals, accountability, and leadership.

I want you to get clear about what you want, and then design backwards to the steps necessary to get there. You are the captain. You have the knowledge and the abilities; you just need to start moving.

We started this book with the fact that leadership will be the most important element to having the practice you've always dreamed about. That very leadership will direct your team, who will be trained to the highest degree and be appreciated for it. They will be the vehicles by which your practice culture is driven.

We went into the importance of life/work balance, and how profitability and efficiency gives you the opportunity to have more of it. The systems and your ability to implement them will be the foundation for the well-oiled dental machine you are about to build.

You should now understand why being clear about your brand to your team and the importance of their understanding of touch points is critical to providing an amazing patient experience consistently day in day out.

We then went into our systems one by one, in hopes that you got some great ideas and made notes about what systems at your office could use a makeover. We know that to have a great practice, we must do more than just "hang our shingle." We need to be intentional about everything we do and why we do it. We need to constantly re-evaluate and communicate with our team to be in a state of constant improvement.

My experience with my practice has been a back and forth journey in which for some weeks, I think we are the greatest practice that was ever created and it no longer needs me to survive, while some weeks I am thinking about how much I can sell it for so that I can do something completely different with my life. Those frustrating moments are the ones that motivate me to get back in there and dissect where we are slipping and get the ship back on course.

Usually those times are when I am spending most of my time enjoying my life outside the practice. You can't be balls to the wall all the time. You just need to be able to realize when the practice growth needs a little more of your personal attention and leadership.

This is the balance between "awesome" and "WTF". As you increase your practice income and profitability, you will have moments where it seems like everything in the world has aligned to make you successful and happy—all the while balanced by periods of decreasing focus and energy and the big killer, the loss of work satisfaction for your team members and yourself.

Dentistry is just like a batting average. You can't be in complete greatness at all times. Don't beat yourself up too much when you are in WTF land.

You need to love what you do, and chances are if you don't, your practice is spending way too much time in WTF. Adjust course and steer your ship. It's possible and it all starts with you.

Butter Cups

I will end on a story I heard from a dental consultant, Loraine Guth. She told a story to me about a restaurant owner who wanted everything at the restaurant to be perfect. He wanted a great environment, great food, impeccable attention to detail, and the best customer service ever.

You know those little butter cups on the table. He wanted those stocked full before the guests were sat at the table. He also wanted the guests to have a friendly connection to the servers. The servers were supposed to make sure the guests were attended to and had a great time.

The owner started noticing that the butter cups weren't getting stocked. He would start walking around, shaming people if they didn't stock their butter cups. One day the restaurant was very slow. One server only had a single table. It was a party of six people and they were having a great time. She made sure she brought their food on time, refilled their drinks, as well as anything else they needed. The table really liked the server and she spent a lot of time just chatting and laughing it up with them.

The guests eventually left and gave her a huge tip. She had

provided excellent service as well as had a great time with them that night.

The owner saw that it was her only table, and noticed that her other tables were lacking butter cups. He was angry. After she finished with her table, he yelled at her, wondering why if she only had one table, she didn't have time to refill the butter cups.

The server was very upset, as she was providing great customer service as the owner had wanted. Yes, her butter cups weren't stocked, but she was busy providing a great experience for her only table.

From that day forward, she stopped spending so much time taking care of her guests and a little more time restocking her butter cups. After all, *that* was really important to the owner and he would let her know when she forgot.

Eventually, the customer service of the entire restaurant began to change, as all the servers learned from experience that the restaurant was not really about great customer service as much as it was about stocked butter cups. Job satisfaction by the servers eventually suffered and the restaurant as a whole, until it finally closed.

What are Your Butter Cups, Doctor?

Never lose sight of what's important in your practice and your life. What are you putting way too much emphasis on, that when you step back and look at it in the big picture, is really not that important? We all have a finite number of "butter cups" that can receive our attention. Everything we focus on takes focus away from something else. Find out what you want out of your practice and your life. Figure out your big picture. Focus on the big things. An unstocked tray of butter cups never hurt anybody. Best of luck to you!

Paul Etchison DDS

Endnotes

1. Kim, M. Julie, Peter C. Damiano, Jed Hand. "Consumer's Choice of Dentists: How and Why People Choose Dental School Faculty Members as Their Oral Health Care Providers." *Journal of Dental Education, 2012.* Vol. 76(6). Pages 695-704. Accessed at http:// scholarscompass.vcu.edu/cgi/viewcontent.cgi? article=1002&context=genp_pubs on 5/22/2017

2. Bureau of Labor Statistics, U.S. Department of Labor, *Occupational Outlook Handbook, 2016-17 Edition,* Dentists, Accessed at https://www.bls.gov/ooh/healthcare/ dentists.htm on 5/22/2017

3. Perry, Mark. "The public thinks the average company makes a 36% profit margin, which is about 5X too high." *AEIdeas: A Public Policy Blog from AEI.* April 2, 2015. Accessed at https://www.aei.org/publication/the-public-thinks-the-average-company-makes-a-36-profit-margin-which-is-about-5x-too-high/ on 5/22/2017

4. Blatchford, Bill. "You Choose Your Overhead." *Dental Economics.* Volume 94, Issue 2. February 1, 2004. Accessed at http://www.dentaleconomics.com/articles/print/volume-94/issue-2/departments/flourishing-in-changing-times/ you-choose-your-overhead.html on 5/22/2017

5. American Association of Endodontists. "Getting to the Root of Dental Phobia." March 29, 2009. Accessed at http://www.aae.org/about-aae/news-room/press-releases/ root-canal-awareness-week-2009.aspx on 7/6/2017

6. Sine, Richard. "Don't Fear the Dentist." *WebMD.* Accessed at http://www.webmd.com/oral-health/features/dont-fear -the-dentist#1 on 5/22/2017

Reading List (Listed in the Order they Appear in the Text)

- Johnson, Spencer. *Who Moved My Cheese: An A-Mazing Way to Deal with Change in Your Work and in Your Life.* G.P. Putnam's Sons. New York: 1998.

- Covey, Stephen R. *The 7 Habits of Highly Effective People: Powerful Lessons in Personal Change.* Simon and Schuster. New York: 2013

- Willink, Jocko and Leif Babin. *Extreme Ownership: How US Navy Seals Lead and Win.* St. Martin's Press. New York: 2015

- Altucher, James. *Altucher Confidential: Ideas for a World Out of Balance.* RTC Publishing. Jacksonville: 2013

- Carnegie, Dale. *How to win Friends and Influence People.* Simon & Schuster. New York: 2010.

- Collins, Jim. *Good to Great: Why Some Companies Make the Leap and Others Don't.* HarperBusiness. New York: 2001.

- Rath, Tom, Mary Reckmeyer, and Maurie J. Manning. *How Full is Your Bucket? For Kids.* Gallup Press. Washington, DC: 2009.

- Joyal, Fred. *Everything is Marketing: The Ultimate Strategy for Dental Practice Growth.* Futuredoctics, 2009.

- Barlow, Janelle and Paul Stewart. *Branded Customer Service: The New Competitive Edge.* Berrett-Koehler Publishers. Oakland, 2006

- Ferriss, Timothy. *The Four Hour Workweek: Escape 9-5, Live Anywhere, and Join the New Rich.* Harmony, 2009.

- Keller, Gary and Jay Papasan. *The ONE Thing: The Surprisingly Simple Truth Behind Extraordinary Results.* Bard Press. Austin: 2013.

- Gerber, Michael E. *The E-Myth Revisited: Why Most Small Businesses Don't Work and What to Do About it.* HarperCollins. New York: 2004.

Made in the USA
Monee, IL
19 March 2021